Living with a Brain Tumor

Living with a
BRAIN TUMOR

Dr. Peter Black's
Guide to
Taking Control
of Your Treatment

◼

Peter Black, M.D., Ph.D.,

with Sharon Cloud Hogan

AN OWL BOOK
Henry Holt and Company   •   New York

Please note that this book is meant to serve as a general guide and is not meant as a substitute for medical care. Patients should seek advice from their own health-care team as well.

In some instances patients' real names were used with permission while others have been changed.

Owl Books
Henry Holt and Company, LLC
Publishers since 1866
175 Fifth Avenue
New York, New York 10010
www.henryholt.com

An Owl Book® and ® are registered trademarks of Henry Holt and Company, LLC.

Distributed in Canada by H. B. Fenn and Company Ltd.

Library of Congress Cataloging-in-Publication Data

Black, Peter.
    Living with a brain tumor : Dr. Peter Black's guide to taking control of your treatment /
Peter Black with Sharon Cloud Hogan.—1st Owl Books ed.
        p.   cm
    ISBN-13: 978-0-8050-7968-5
    ISBN-10: 0-8050-7968-8
    1. Brain—Tumors—Popular works.   I. Hogan, Sharon Cloud.   II. Title.

RC280.B7B53 2006
616.99'481—dc22   2006048259

Henry Holt books are available for special promotions
and premiums. For details contact: Director, Special Markets.

Excerpt from *Autobiography of a Face* by Lucy Grealy. Copyright © 1994 by Lucy Grealy. Reprinted by permission of Houghton Mifflin Company. All rights reserved. "Do Not Go Gentle into That Good Night" by Dylan Thomas, from *The Poems of Dylan Thomas*, copyright © 1952 by Dylan Thomas. Reprinted by permission of New Directions Publishing Corp. Excerpts from Ivan Noble's blog, "Tumour Diary." Courtesy of BBC News Online. Excerpts from *An Open Approach to Living with Cancer* by John Calvin Hammock. Copyright © 2004 by John Calvin Hammock. Reprinted by permission of John Calvin Hammock. "Table 1. Summary of Targeted Therapies for Malignant Glioma." Reprinted by permission of *Current Medicine* publication. Excerpts from *I Had Brain Surgery, What's Your Excuse?* by Suzanne Becker. Copyright © 2004 by Suzanne Becker. Reprinted by permission of Workman Publishing Co., Inc. All rights reserved. "The Peace of Wild Things" by Wendell Berry, from *Collected Poems, 1957–1982*, copyright © 1985 by Wendell Berry. Reprinted by permission of North Point, Farrar, Straus and Giroux, LLC.

First Owl Books Edition 2006

Designed by Victoria Hartman

Printed in the United States of America

1   3   5   7   9   10   8   6   4   2

For patients with brain tumors,
their families, and their friends

CONTENTS

———■———

Part Four: Treatment Options

Part Five: Recovery

PREFACE

———————————————■———————————————

Ann, an attractive thirty-year-old woman with two children, is sitting in my office on a beautiful autumn day. We have just discovered that she has a brain tumor. She is stunned; her face betrays fear and hopelessness as the panic mounts inside her. I try to reassure her by explaining that her tumor is probably benign, that almost half of all tumors originating in the brain are benign. But I can sense that, in her shock, Ann has not really heard my words or does not really believe them. For her, "brain tumor" means death or major disability.

Every year in the United States, more than 100,000 people like Ann face the unexpected diagnosis of a brain tumor. Approximately 40,000 of these tumors originate in the brain; the rest have spread from cancers in the lung, colon, breast, or elsewhere in the body. Malignant brain tumors are the second leading cause of cancer death in children and in adults younger than age 34, and they are a major cause of disability in men and women in their fifties and sixties. They are the second-fastest-growing cause of cancer death among people over age 65, behind lung cancer.

As a practicing neurosurgeon for more than twenty-five years, I have cared for more than 5,000 patients with brain tumors. One of the first things my patients want to know when they're diagnosed with a brain tumor is how that tumor is going to affect their lives, their ability to pursue their normal activities, and their relationships with loved ones. Every week, when I counsel patients like Ann, I wish that I could refer them to an up-to-date, accurate, comprehensive book about what they are going through. Remarkably, there are very few current books on this subject for readers who are not medical professionals.

I want people with brain tumors to know that many kinds of brain tumors are compatible with a long and productive life. If you have a brain tumor, I want you to know you are not alone. I want to get the word out that many people do survive a brain tumor for many years, and even with the tumors that remain difficult to treat, we've made promising inroads. If more people know about brain tumors, our scientific funding agencies may support more investigations into their cause and treatment. This book is meant for brain tumor patients; for their families and friends; and for the doctors, nurses, and mental health professionals who treat, comfort, and advise them.

PART ONE

—■—

An Introduction
to Brain Tumors

I have a recurring dream of a large gathering of all the brain tumor patients I have ever seen. At least half the people in my dream are patients who have lived with (or without!) their tumor for ten years or more. Most of them are so normal in appearance and action that you would never know they've had a tumor. Another group, comprised of those who had tumors in early childhood or adolescence, might show some characteristic long-term effects of their tumor. About 20 percent would have a definite problem with movement, memory, or behavior as a result of their tumor treatment. Finally, about 10 percent are clearly struggling every day with an uncertain future and the effects of their tumor and its treatment. All of these former patients are, however, united by one crucial fact—their lives have been changed forever by their experiences with their brain tumor.

If you or someone you know has been diagnosed with a brain tumor, it is important not to panic until you know more. In Part One, I will describe what a brain tumor is, how it grows, and what it does to the brain. I also will explain how doctors diagnose a brain tumor. In Part Two, you will find a guide to the different types of brain tumors. Parts Three and Four contain information about living with brain tumors and the many different treatment options that are available. The last part of the book, Part Five, suggests a number of ways to work toward wellness and the many reasons why you should never give up hope.

1

■

What Is a Brain Tumor?

A brain tumor is a mass of abnormal cells growing in the brain. The cells can come from the brain itself, from its lining, or from other places in the body. Brain tumors that develop in the brain itself (from brain cells, blood vessels, nerves, or membranes covering the brain) are called *primary brain tumors*. They may be benign or malignant. *Benign brain tumors* grow slowly and do not invade brain tissue; examples are meningiomas, vestibular schwannomas, and pituitary adenomas. They still pose a threat to health because they may put pressure on important areas of the brain. *Malignant primary brain tumors* spread into the healthy tissues that surround them and tend to grow more quickly than benign tumors. They are difficult to treat because they spread into the brain like alien invaders in a population of normal citizens.

Brain tumors that spread from cancer elsewhere in the body (such as skin, breast, lung, or colon cancer) are *secondary* or *metastatic brain tumors*. They are all malignant.

What Causes a Brain Tumor? Why Me?

If you or your friend or family member has been diagnosed with a brain tumor, you may ask what you did wrong to deserve it. It's important to remember that a brain tumor is not your fault. In most cases, it's random—something we don't know how to prevent. It's not your cell phone. It's not because of something you ate or didn't eat. It's not a punishment for something that you may have done in the past. Although we know some factors that are associated with brain tumors, altogether they account for fewer than 10 percent of the tumors we see. These factors include genes, radiation, and some chemicals. But in most cases, we simply don't understand what causes these tumors.

In this section I will discuss briefly what we do know about the factors associated with brain tumors. You might want to know that epidemiologists—researchers who investigate the incidence and control of disease in a given population—are working very hard to determine which environmental and other factors may set the stage for brain tumors. Their research will be increasingly important in the future.

Genetic Disorders

Table 1-1 lists some genetic disorders that are associated with brain tumors.

TABLE 1-1

Genetic disorders associated with brain tumors

Disorder	Relevance to Brain Tumors
Neurofibromatosis 1 (also called Von Recklinghausen's disease)	Causes soft tumors all over the body; there may be nervous system tumors as well.
Neurofibromatosis 2	Leads to tumors mainly within the nervous system; these may include schwannomas, astrocytomas, and meningiomas. (The different types of tumors are discussed in chapter 3.)
Turcot's syndrome	Causes polyps on the colon. This syndrome has been linked with glioblastomas and medulloblastomas.
Li-Fraumeni syndrome	This rare inherited syndrome is associated with several malignant familial tumors including glioblastoma.

Disorder	Relevance to Brain Tumors
Gorlin's syndrome	Predisposes people to skin lesions.
Hereditary nonpolyposis colorectal cancer (HNPCC)	People with this type of cancer are prone to high-grade gliomas.
Tuberous sclerosis	May be associated with a benign kind of astrocytoma in an area of the brain called the ventricle.

Additional genetic factors may predispose certain people to cancer. Sixteen percent of patients with primary brain tumors have a family history of cancer. This has led to the concept of cancer susceptibility genes—genes that by themselves do not cause cancer but make it more likely that a cancer will develop. Scientists are presently sorting out what these genes are and how they cause tumors.

Radiation

Past radiation to the head and neck may cause astrocytomas, meningiomas, and some other tumors. These "radiation-induced" tumors occur five to twenty years after the original irradiation; we think they occur because of DNA damage sustained during prolonged radiation therapy. There is no evidence that the small amounts of radiation from diagnostic x-rays cause brain tumors.

Chemical Exposure and Diet

Exposure to certain chemicals such as vinyl chloride, N-nitrosourea compounds, and some pesticides (which are no longer on the market) may lead to astrocytomas. Tobacco, alcohol, and diet have not been directly associated with brain tumors.

Electromagnetic Fields

Some researchers and patients have raised concerns about a link between brain tumors and the electromagnetic fields (EMFs) surrounding cell phones or high-tension wires. Several recent studies have shown no such correlation.

Head Injury

There is no convincing evidence that head trauma causes brain tumors.

How Does a Brain Tumor Develop?

A brain tumor appears to come from one abnormal brain cell that grows when it is not supposed to. At least five changes allow it to develop. One change is that the cell learns to stimulate its own growth by producing growth factors that encourage its division. These growth factors are the product of genes called oncogenes. When they are turned on in the cell, they stimulate growth of that cell and the cells around it. We don't know why these genes are turned on, however.

A second change is that a tumor cell may lose "tumor suppressor genes." The cell uses these genes to divide during development, but then they normally are turned off. An example is the gene called merlin that is lost or defective in a condition called neurofibromatosis; as a result of this, cells continue to grow.

Third, malignant tumor cells learn to spread into the brain by dissolving the matrix of brain tissue and traveling through it; this process is called *invasion*.

Fourth, primary malignant tumors may hide themselves from the normal immune cells of the brain by coating themselves with molecules that make them invisible.

Last, malignant tumors may form new blood vessels in order to increase their own nutrient supply and enhance growth. This process is called *angiogenesis*.

Our understanding of these possible causes of brain tumor growth is important because it may help us to treat brain tumors by blocking growth factors with "smart" drugs, by replacing defective tumor suppressor genes with gene therapy, by preventing invasion, by enhancing the immune response, or by blocking new blood vessel formation. We will discuss all of these new therapies in chapter 14.

What Does a Brain Tumor Do to the Brain?

*If the human brain were so simple that we could understand it, we
would be so simple that we couldn't.*

—Scientist Emerson M. Pugh

Now that we've run through the mechanics of brain tumors, let's take a
look at how they affect the brain. The first step is to give you a brief
anatomy lesson about the brain, its component parts and what they do, so
you can understand how a tumor affects the way a normal brain functions.
Some parts of your body can expand and contract because only skin covers them. The enlarging waist is a problem for your clothes, but not for
your body. The brain is different because it lives inside the skull and the
skull cannot enlarge to accommodate anything more than the structures it
already houses: the brain, cerebrospinal fluid, and blood vessels. A brain
tumor is a mass that is an unwelcome addition that presses on important
brain parts. Here is an introduction to these parts and what they do.

Cerebrum

Where it is: The cerebrum, the largest part of your brain, occupies the
upper two-thirds of your head. It contains a right and a left hemisphere
connected by the *corpus callosum,* which sends messages from one side of
the brain to the other. The cerebrum also contains the basal ganglia, thalamus, and lateral and third ventricles.

What it's made of: Most of the cerebrum is made up of glial cells (astrocytes, oligodendrocytes, or ependymal cells), whose functions are poorly
understood. About 5 percent of cerebral cells are neurons, which transmit
nerve impulses. These cells make up the gray matter, the outer part of the
brain. The central part of the cerebrum is composed of fibers that connect
the cerebrum to the rest of the brain. There are four lobes in the cerebrum:
frontal, parietal, temporal, and occipital (see figure 1).

What happens there: The cerebrum is the source of conscious activity.
It controls sensation, movement, hearing, and vision. The right hemisphere directs the left side of the body and the left hemisphere controls the
right side.

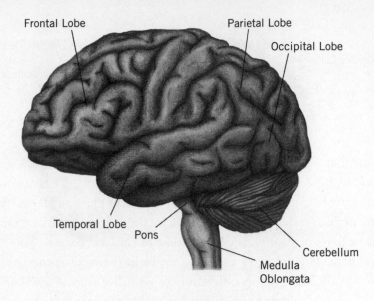

Frontal Lobe

Parietal Lobe

Occipital Lobe

Temporal Lobe

Pons

Cerebellum

Medulla
Oblongata

Figure 1.   The major components of the brain.

Frontal Lobe

Where it is: Your frontal lobe begins just behind your forehead and extends halfway back in your skull.

What happens there: The frontal lobe contributes to bodily movement, speech, decision making, planning, reasoning, personality, creativity, mood, and inhibition.

Parietal Lobe

Where it is: The parietal lobe sits at the top of your head, behind the frontal lobe.

What happens there: The parietal lobe controls your sense of touch and some of your visual capacity, including your ability to recognize what you see.

Temporal Lobe

Where it is: Your temporal lobe is below your frontal and parietal lobes, just above your ear.

What happens there: This part of your brain is important in hearing and may also affect speech, behavior, emotions, and memory.

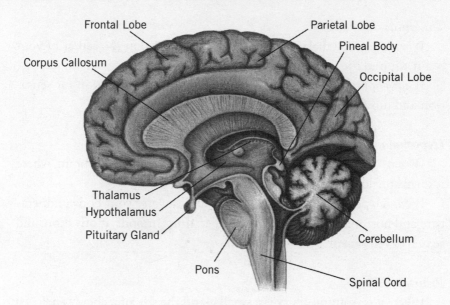

Frontal Lobe

Parietal Lobe

Pineal Body

Corpus Callosum

Occipital Lobe

Thalamus

Hypothalamus

Pituitary Gland

Cerebellum

Pons

Spinal Cord

Figure 2.

A sagittal (sideways) section of the middle portion of the brain showing the thalamus, hypothalamus, and pituitary gland.

Occipital Lobe

Where it is: The occipital lobe is located in the back of your head.

What happens there: This part of the brain is important in vision.

Ventricles

Where they are: Deep inside the cerebrum are the "great lakes" of the brain—four cerebral ventricles that form the brain's *ventricular system*. These ventricles are filled with a clear liquid called cerebrospinal fluid (CSF) in which the brain floats. Sometimes a brain tumor blocks the flow of CSF and these "lakes" overflow—this condition, called hydrocephalus, can be life-threatening.

Basal Ganglia

Where they are: The basal ganglia include the putamen and the globus pallidus. They are deep inside the cerebrum and form the walls of the lateral ventricles.

What they do: The basal ganglia are important in the smoothness of movement.

Thalamus

Where it is: The thalamus (see figure 2)is located at the center of your brain, around the third ventricle.

What happens there: Your thalamus serves as a relay station for sensation and movement.

Hypothalamus

Where it is: The hypothalamus is located deep inside your brain, where it forms the lower wall of the third ventricle.

What happens there: Your hypothalamus regulates your body temperature and hormones. It affects your hunger, thirst, moods, motivation, and sexual development.

Pituitary Gland

Where it is: Your pituitary is a small gland the size of a cherry enclosed in the bony *sella turcica* (which translates as "Turkish saddle") at the base of the brain. It is connected to your hypothalamus and is composed of two lobes: the anterior lobe (*adenohypophysis*) and the posterior lobe (*neurohypophysis*).

What happens there: The pituitary gland is a master hormonal gland that controls the thyroid and adrenal glands and the sexual organs. It also controls water balance in the body.

Cerebellum

Where it is: The cerebellum is the second largest part of your brain. It is located in the back of your head just above your neck, and it covers the brain stem at the base of your brain. Like the cerebrum, the cerebellum has two hemispheres; the right cerebellum controls the right side of the body.

What happens there: Your cerebellum controls your balance, coordination, and fine-muscle movement. There is increasing evidence that it has cognitive effects as well.

Brain Stem

Where it is: The brain stem is at the base of the brain, protected by the cerebrum and cerebellum. This part of your brain, which is composed of the *midbrain, pons,* and *medulla oblongata,* connects the cerebrum to the spinal cord.

What happens there: Your vital physical functions like breathing, eye movements, swallowing, heartbeat, and blood pressure are all controlled from the brain stem. In particular, the reticular formation is responsible for consciousness and patterns of sleeping and eating. The midbrain is related to hearing and sight. The pons conveys impulses between the largest parts of your brain—the cerebrum and cerebellum—and your spinal cord.

Pineal Gland

Where it is: This gland is just beneath the corpus callosum, behind the third ventricle.

What happens there: Your pineal gland regulates sleep and other body rhythms.

Meninges

Where they are: Three sheets of tissue called the meninges surround the brain. The first of these sheets is the *pia,* which tightly surrounds the cerebrum and cerebellum. The second is the *arachnoid,* which is more loosely connected to the skull and contains CSF. The third is the *dura,* a very tough outer layer that is tightly connected to the skull.

What happens there: The dura divides the brain compartments into three sections—*the falx* separates the right and left hemispheres of the cerebrum and the *tentorium* separates the cerebrum from the cerebellum. The dura also has several large venous channels called sinuses, which are important exit routes for blood. Meningiomas are brain tumors that grow from the meninges.

Cranial Nerves

Cranial nerves (see figure 3) connect your brain to the sensation and movement components of your face. Here is a table of their names and functions:

TABLE 1-2

Cranial Nerves

No.	Name	What It controls
I	Olfactory	Smell
II	Optic	Sight

No.	Name	What It controls
III	Oculomotor	Pupil size, some movements of the eyes and upper eyelid movement
IV	Trochlear	Some movements of the eyes (down and in)
V	Trigeminal	Facial and mouth sensation; chewing muscles
VI	Abducens	Eye movements sideways
VII	Facial	Facial movement, taste, secretion of saliva and tears
VIII	Vestibulocochlear	Hearing and balance
IX	Glossopharyngeal	Sensation and movement in the throat, taste (back of the tongue)
X	Vagus	Feeling in the throat and windpipe; organs in the abdomen and chest (heart, lungs, bowels, stomach); throat and windpipe muscles
XI	Accessory	Neck movement
XII	Hypoglossal	Movement of the tongue, swallowing

Other Terms You May Hear

Blood brain barrier. A mechanism by which the blood vessels of the brain filter out and prevent substances in the blood from reaching the brain. This protects the brain from the chemicals in the blood.

Descending tract. Nerves that descend from the brain to the spinal cord.

Glia. Most of the tissue of the brain is composed of *glial cells.* These cells may be either *astrocytes,* star-shaped cells that are crucial to metabolism in the brain; *oligodendrocytes,* which maintain myelin over the nerve cells and help them communicate with each other; or *ependymal cells,* which line the ventricles of the brain. Most brain tumors originate from glial cells.

Tentorium. The tentorium is a flap of dura that creates a sort of horizontal dividing line between the top and bottom of the brain. The upper area above the tentorium (which includes the cerebral hemispheres) is called the *supratentorial compartment.* Most brain tumors in adults are *supratentorial.* The bottom section of the brain, which is made up of both the cerebellum and the brain stem, is called the *infratentorial compartment* (or *posterior fossa*). Most brain tumors in children are *infratentorial.*

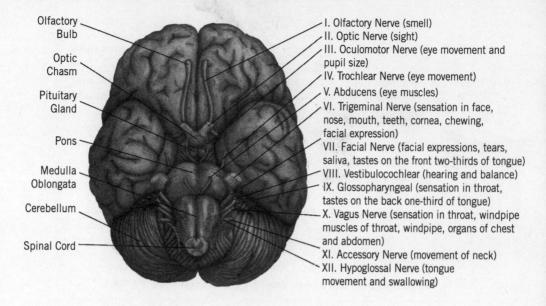

Olfactory Bulb
Optic Chasm
Pituitary Gland
Pons
Medulla Oblongata
Cerebellum
Spinal Cord

I. Olfactory Nerve (smell)
II. Optic Nerve (sight)
III. Oculomotor Nerve (eye movement and pupil size)
IV. Trochlear Nerve (eye movement)
V. Abducens (eye muscles)
VI. Trigeminal Nerve (sensation in face, nose, mouth, teeth, cornea, chewing, facial expression)
VII. Facial Nerve (facial expressions, tears, saliva, tastes on the front two-thirds of tongue)
VIII. Vestibulocochlear (hearing and balance)
IX. Glossopharyngeal (sensation in throat, tastes on the back one-third of tongue)
X. Vagus Nerve (sensation in throat, windpipe muscles of throat, windpipe, organs of chest and abdomen)
XI. Accessory Nerve (movement of neck)
XII. Hypoglossal Nerve (tongue movement and swallowing)

Figure 3.   The cranial nerves.

A view from the base of the brain showing the
cranial nerves and other brain structures.

Cranium. Another word for the skull. The cranium includes the ethnoid, frontal, sphenoid, temporal, parietal, and occipital bones.

Skull base. The bones at the bottom of the skull, beneath the frontal and temporal lobes, the cerebellum, and the brain stem.

Now that you know what a brain tumor is, how it grows, and what it does to the brain, let's move on to chapter 2, where I will explain how we diagnose brain tumors.

2

---■---

How Brain Tumors Are Diagnosed

*Our son kept sitting closer and closer to the TV. We thought it was
just his prescription for glasses—how did we know it was a brain
tumor pressing on his optic nerves?*
                                    —Mother of a child with a brain tumor

*I hit my head and had a CT scan—the next thing I knew a doctor
was telling me I had a brain tumor. How weird is that?*
                                    —Brain tumor patient

He was fine and then he wasn't fine.
                                    —Father of a child with a brain tumor

In the early twentieth century, a doctor named Harvey Cushing started the
surgical specialty of neurosurgery. Working at the Peter Bent Brigham
Hospital in Boston, Cushing demonstrated that a neurosurgeon could
operate on brain tumors safely. At that time, the only way to diagnose
brain tumors was to listen to a patient's story, do a physical examination,
and evaluate skull x-ray films.

Three generations later, much has changed. The Peter Bent Brigham
Hospital has become Brigham and Women's Hospital, a major teaching
hospital of Harvard Medical School. More than 20,000 neurosurgeons
worldwide perform neurosurgery for brain tumors, blood vessel abnormalities, spine problems, pediatric diseases, movement disorders, epilepsy,
and pain. Brain tumor imaging also has been considerably improved. With
magnetic resonance imaging (MRI), we can image the brain, its blood vessels, and its tracts without invading the body. With a positron emission

tomographic (PET) or single-photon emission computed tomographic (SPECT) scan, we can assess metabolic activity; with an electroencephalogram (EEG) or evoked potential we can analyze electrical signals in the nervous system. In this chapter, I will describe some of the remarkable techniques we now have to diagnose a brain tumor and to determine what kind it might be. First, though, let's look at some of the reasons why patients and physicians might suspect a brain tumor.

Possible Symptoms and Signs of a Brain Tumor

Headaches, weakness, vision loss, hearing loss, unsteadiness, seizures, and other problems may all be indicators of a brain tumor. Ten years ago, it was painful and sometimes dangerous to do the studies that could assess whether there was actually a tumor underlying these symptoms. These are common complaints and usually don't mean that a person necessarily has a brain tumor. Imaging can distinguish some of these conditions from brain tumors; others require a biopsy. Table 2-1 lists some of the conditions that can resemble a brain tumor.

Fortunately, we have advanced remarkably in our ability to diagnose brain tumors without invading the body. CT, MRI, and PET scans have completely changed our capacity to make an efficient and accurate diagnosis. In this chapter, I will tell you about these diagnostic tools.

TABLE 2-1

Conditions That May Mimic a Brain Tumor

Condition	What Distinguishes It from a Tumor
Benign intracranial hypertension (causes headaches and high brain pressure)	MRI scan
Brain abscess (infection that creates a mass that looks like a tumor)	Biopsy
Brain cyst (a fluid-filled mass)	MRI scan
Central nervous system (CNS) vasculitis (blood vessel inflammation)	Biopsy
Hamartoma (abnormality formed at birth)	Biopsy

Condition	What Distinguishes It from a Tumor
Hydrocephalus (may cause headaches and high brain pressure)	MRI
Multiple sclerosis (may be associated with an abnormal brain mass)	MRI or biopsy
Progressive multifocal leukoencephalopathy	Biopsy
Stroke (may look like a tumor on MRI)	MRI or biopsy
Subdural hematoma (may cause headaches)	MRI
Vascular malformation	MRI (usually)

What makes us suspect that a patient may have a tumor? As doctors, we talk about "symptoms" and "signs." The word *symptom* comes from the Greek *symptoma,* which means "something that befalls you." A symptom is something that you as a patient feel and describe as being abnormal. A sign, in contrast, is a change that is evident to another person.

Brain tumors cause a number of symptoms and signs, depending on the type of tumor and its location. Sometimes they cause no symptoms at all; an MRI or CT scan done for some other reason may reveal a brain mass. Other symptoms may be as mild as a slight headache or as severe as a seizure or stroke.

Some symptoms and signs that might suggest a brain tumor are:

Headaches that wake you up in the middle of the night and are more severe in the morning. They may be worse if you change position, cough, or exercise and are usually different from headaches you might commonly experience. Nausea and vomiting may accompany them.

Persistent nausea and vomiting, especially when associated with a headache. These are signs of increased pressure in the head.

Seizures (convulsions) are sudden movements or sensations caused by abnormal electrical impulses in the brain (see box, pp. 20–21). A generalized (*grand mal*) seizure involves loss of consciousness and shaking of the arms or legs. A simple or partial (*petit mal* or *absence*) seizure affects a person's consciousness briefly. A *focal* seizure involves one arm or leg. A *partial complex* seizure may involve repeated automatic movements. Any of these signs may suggest a brain tumor, and a first-time seizure in an adult should be investigated by a CT or MRI scan.

Weakness, loss of sensation, or numbness; unsteadiness or lack of coordination when walking (ataxia); or muscular weakness on one side of the body (hemiparesis) are signs of pressure on a specific part of the brain.

Hearing loss can be caused by a brain tumor called a *vestibular schwannoma* (also called an *acoustic neuroma*). This type of sensorineural hearing loss differs from conductive hearing loss in that it cannot be corrected with a hearing aid.

Loss of vision in one or both eyes may be caused by a tumor pressing on the optic nerve itself or by a tumor in the visual pathways. Double vision (*diplopia*) may occur with tumors that press on the nerves of eye movement or the brain stem.

Speech difficulties may include loss of the ability to write, speak, or understand words. A person may have either difficulty forming words (*aphasia*) or difficulty articulating them (*dysarthria*).

Other problems that may suggest a brain tumor include *trouble concentrating, confusion, and difficulty finding one's way; memory loss; extreme drowsiness; and a dramatic change in behavior or a sudden loss of interest in usual activities.*

In women, *menstrual periods may stop abnormally (amenorrhea)* and some women with pituitary tumors may not be able to get pregnant. Men with pituitary tumors may lose their sex drive.

Most of these symptoms and signs are not specific to a brain tumor, and most people who have them do not have tumors. If you are experiencing one or more of these symptoms, tell your doctor. If the symptoms continue, request an MRI. If a diagnostic scan does reveal a brain tumor, the sooner you receive treatment, the better.

> *My primary care doctor looked upon me as a hypochondriac and treated me as possibly depressed. Just prior to the discovery of my meningioma, my doctor had basically given up and was prescribing health food remedies. One reason I wasn't taken seriously was that I always saved my sick days for my children's emergencies that could arise throughout the year. Because I was still showing up for work, even when feeling very ill, my doctor assumed I was not as sick as my complaints would indicate.*
>
> *I began to feel that my doctor might be right; everyone has aches and pains, so I just needed to tough it out. As time passed, this became more and more difficult. After the fact, and now*

looking back, I didn't place enough emphasis on my headaches. I thought they were a product of my earlier encephalitis; therefore, I didn't have an MRI performed until they became constant and unbearable.

—Patient with a meningioma

This is not an unusual story, because brain tumors may have very subtle manifestations. One of my patients was treated for a year for symptoms of "menopause," such as mild headaches and easy distractability, before a tumor was finally diagnosed. Another patient, who turned out to have a tumor called an acoustic neuroma, was told that her dizziness and the ringing that she heard in her right ear were due to stress. Her tumor was only discovered when an ear, nose, and throat (ENT) doctor did a hearing test and then sent her for an MRI scan. Time and time again my patients have said that they knew that something was wrong, but the first doctor they went to attributed their symptoms to depression, stress, or another unrelated health problem. If you are convinced something is wrong, try to get a CT or an MRI scan. It cannot be stressed enough: the sooner we diagnose a brain tumor, the sooner it can be treated.

Seizures

What are they? Who gets them? People with brain tumors may experience seizures. These temporary electrical storms in the brain may last just a minute or two, but the recovery from them can last longer.

A *partial seizure* begins in one part of the brain's cortex. If the patient remains conscious, it is called a *simple partial seizure*—it may, for example, involve the shaking of an arm or leg. A partial seizure during which the person loses consciousness is called a *complex partial seizure.*

A *generalized seizure* involves the entire brain, and the patient loses consciousness. This type of seizure may be generalized in one area from the beginning or may involve secondary generalization when the seizure spreads from one area to other areas of the brain. During this form of seizure, the person may pass out for a minute or two. His or her arms and legs may have jerky (tonic-clonic) movements. Seizures that continue over and over again may lead to a dangerous condition called *status epilepticus.*

How are seizures diagnosed? We diagnose seizures through a description of the seizure by another person who witnessed it. An EEG provides important confirmation. Sometimes we have to distinguish seizures from other problems such as a sleep disorder, a mini-stroke (*transient ischemic attack*), migraine headaches, or fainting.

How are seizures treated? Therapy with anti-seizure (also called anti-convulsant) drugs is most often effective in managing seizures that are associated with brain tumors. These drugs include: phenytoin (Dilantin); carbamazepine (Tegretol, Carbatrol); oxcarbazepine (Trileptal); phenobarbital; valproic acid (Depakote); gabapentin (Neurontin); lamotrigine (Lamictal); tiagabine (Gabitril); topiramate (Topamax); zonisamide (Zonegran); levetiracetam (Keppra); and pregabalin (Lyrica). I will explain more about these drugs in chapter 15.

Talk with the physician who is prescribing these drugs for you before you begin to take them. Some anticonvulsant medications can interact poorly with other drugs you may be taking, such as birth control pills and an anti-inflammatory medication called dexamethasone. If your doctor prescribes anticonvulsant drugs, you may begin taking them at low doses and gradually increase the dosages until your seizures are well controlled. The side effects of these medicines may include sleepiness and dizziness.

Sometimes surgery to remove at least part of the tumor can help to control seizures. A vagus nerve stimulator, a device that is implanted in the chest and emits electrical impulses, can also be helpful for some people.

Getting plenty of rest and relaxation can also help control seizures. Talking with a counselor or neurologist about the effects of seizures on your life may be helpful in dealing with them.

The Visit with the Doctor

If you think you have symptoms that suggest a brain tumor, make an appointment with your doctor. You may wish to take a friend or family member with you for support, and to help you remember the doctor's advice. You should be prepared to give your physician the following information (it is often helpful to write this information down beforehand):

- The nature and duration of your symptoms, and what (if anything) has made them worse or better
- Other health problems you may have had, including cancer
- Past surgery and any complications related to it
- Medications you are taking and how often you take them
- Allergies to any drugs or other compounds

The doctor may perform several tests besides the usual physical exam to figure out if a brain tumor may be the cause behind your symptoms. These may include vision tests to assess your eye movements; the reactions of your pupils; and, with an ophthalmoscope, to detect *papilledema*, swelling behind your eyes caused by increased pressure in the brain. He or she will also evaluate your sense of smell, hearing, facial movements, and speech. Your doctor will check your reflexes, balance, movement, and coordination (for instance, he or she may ask you to quickly touch your nose with your finger tip or walk in a straight line). The examination also may include a test called the Mini-Mental Status Examination (MMSE) to evaluate your memory and orientation.

If your doctor suspects a brain tumor or other serious cause of your trouble, he or she may ask for other tests including brain imaging and function tests. Think about asking your doctor or the imaging center for a CD with your images on it. It may help you to understand your problem better if you go over the pictures with your physician.

Brain Imaging

> The scan itself is not unpleasant apart from the injection halfway through (a contrast agent to make the tumor more visible). But the results need writing up by a specialist and sending on to my doctor, which usually takes two days and leaves plenty of time for nerves to fray.
>
> —Ivan Noble, BBC reporter

Brain imaging has remarkably improved our ability to diagnose brain tumors. In this section, I will explain which types of scans are available to help determine what type of tumor you may have.

Skull X-Ray Films

Skull x-ray films are not very useful for diagnosing a brain tumor, but they may show calcification in a tumor or an enlarged bony structure at the skull base called the *sella turcica* (Turkish saddle); this enlarged area may suggest a pituitary tumor.

CT Scan

Computed tomographic (CT) scanning uses traditional x-rays to pick up subtle differences in tissue. This type of scan displays the brain in cross section. With the injection of a type of dye called a contrast agent, it can show some malignant tumors very clearly.

How Does It Work? The CT machine rotates around your head and passes many thin x-ray beams through it. The brain and skull absorb the radiation and the density is in turn conveyed back to a computer, which builds enhanced, cross-sectional images of the brain. The most dense structures (such as the skull, a tumor, or a blood clot) appear white and the least dense structures (such as cerebrospinal fluid) appear dark.

CT imaging may be done both with and without the injection of an iodine-based contrast agent. In this "enhanced" scan, the contrast enters leaky blood vessels in a tumor and allows us to see the tumor mass directly, especially if the mass has a rich blood supply. On an enhanced CT scan, glioblastomas, abscesses, and metastatic brain tumors may appear to be encircled by a white ring. It may be difficult to tell them apart without a tissue biopsy.

What Does It Feel Like? During a CT scan, you will lie on a table that moves into a machine that has a round opening. This scanning machine will rotate around your head, sending x-rays toward your brain from several directions. The scanner does not make much sound and you will not be able to feel the x-rays. The opening in the machine is quite large and the scan usually takes twenty minutes or less. The room may be chilly, so we usually advise patients to wear a sweater.

If your imaging will involve a contrast agent, a few scans will generally be taken first and then the dye will be injected into your arm during additional scans. If you are allergic to shellfish, let the radiologist know, because some contrast agents contain iodine.

How Soon Will I Know the Results? A neuroradiologist (a doctor with special training in reading images of the brain) will usually report on your CT scan within 24 hours.

Terms you may read in the CT report:

- *Isodense:* having the same density as brain tissue
- *Hypodense:* having less density than brain tissue
- *Hyperintense:* having greater density than brain tissue

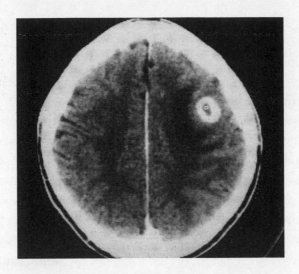

Figure 2-1. A CT scan of a left frontal mass.

The mass was thought to be a malignant tumor (note that the left side of a CT is the right side of the brain). This mass turned out to be a brain abscess, a curable infection that is sometimes hard to distinguish from a tumor.

MRI

Magnetic resonance imaging (MRI) has been available since the 1980s. This preferred test for looking at a brain tumor places the brain in a strong magnetic field and reveals the movement of water in the brain tissue.

How Does It Work? Instead of x-rays (used in CT scans), MRIs make use of a magnetic field. Imagine that the hydrogen molecules in your brain are soldiers. When your head is inside an MRI scanner, those soldiers are on duty. A powerful magnet inside the MRI scanner makes them "line up" and stand at attention. Next, the MRI machine brings in a "commander"— it emits radio energy from a radio coil that instructs the atoms to change direction. They do. Then the radio signal stops and the soldiers are "at ease"—they can relax and go back to their original state. Whenever the molecules/soldiers move around, they give off energy (resonance) in the form of an electromagnetic signal. Atoms from both good and bad soldiers—healthy and diseased cells—have different signals; a computer reads them and converts them into an image.

MRI scanning does not use radiation and it allows physicians to view three-dimensional images of the tumor from various angles. Just as with

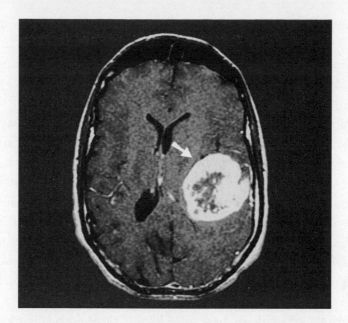

Figure 2-2. An MRI scan of a glioblastoma.

The arrow points to the left temporal glioblastoma. It is white because of leaking of intravenous contrast into the tumor mass from blood vessels. The dark center contains dead tissue.

CT scans, contrast agents (usually an agent called gadolinium) can be used to delineate certain lesions. The MRI contrast is not iodine based, so it does not create problems if you are allergic to shellfish. These dyes are usually injected into the arm during the scanning process.

People who have pacemakers, cardiac monitors, or other metallic implanted devices cannot have an MRI.

Newer MRI techniques that you may encounter are:

- *Diffusion tensor MRI:* shows the fiber tracts of the brain.
- *Echo planar MRI (also called real-time MRI, fast MRI, or functional MRI):* reveals brain function by showing small changes in blood flow.
- *Magnetic resonance angiography (MRA):* shows the blood vessels of the brain.
- *Magnetic resonance spectroscopy (MRS):* provides information about a tumor's metabolism.

What Does It Feel Like? Before an MRI scan, you will need to take off all metal jewelry, hair clips, an underwire bra, and other objects that contain metal. Because you cannot wear pants that have metal grommets, we advise our patients to wear sweatpants instead of jeans.

The room with the MRI machine may be cold, so you may want to wear warm clothing. During an MRI, the table slides all the way into a tube-like machine. Although the idea of entering this type of machine may make you uneasy, remember that you will be able to communicate with the technician during the scan. The test is painless, and the only challenging part is that you must remain still for a while. If you tend to get claustrophobic or anxious, tell your doctor. You may be able to take a mild sedative (like Ativan) before your MRI, but we cannot put you to sleep completely because you will need to stay awake during the test. Some patients find it helpful to take some deep breaths to relax. Children may imagine that they are lying in a space capsule.

During the test, you will hear some loud clicking and clanging sounds. The test usually lasts about 45 minutes. You might want to bring your own earplugs (or ask the MRI technician for some) to lessen the sound. If it helps, pretend that you're at a rock concert. You may also bring a tape or CD of music with you to the appointment and the technician can pipe it into the MRI room while you are having your scan.

Instead of the closed MRI machine, some patients have an "open" MRI. Rather than a tunnel-like device that you have to physically enter, an open MRI is more like lying on a bridge. Although this is more appealing if you tend to get claustrophobic, an open MRI does not provide as clear a picture as a conventional MRI.

How Soon Will I Know the Results? Just as with CT scans, a neuroradiologist, who specializes in interpreting scans of the brain, will read these images. You will most likely have the results within 48 hours.

Terms you may read in an MRI report:

- *Artifact:* Images on an MRI scan that may be caused by the movement of the person during the scan, metal, or a processing problem.
- *Increased signal:* Objects that appear to be whiter than surrounding areas on an MRI scan.
- *Decreased signal:* Objects that appear to be darker than surrounding areas on an MRI scan.

- *Sagittal image:* A sideways MRI image that splits the brain into left and right sections; this type of image is useful for revealing tumors in the center of the brain.
- *Coronal image:* An MRI image that splits the brain into front and back sections; these anterior-posterior images are useful for revealing tumors deep inside the brain.
- *Enhanced MRI:* An MRI after contrast is given. The contrast most often used is gadolinium, which is not iodine-based but works like the contrast used with CT—it shows up in leaky tissue.
- *FLAIR sequence:* A way of doing an MRI that is particularly sensitive to water in the brain; it is good for telling whether there is swelling (edema) around a tumor.
- *Proton density:* The number of molecules of water in the nuclear signals that an MRI scan picks up in a particular area.
- *T1-weighted:* The time needed for the body's hydrogen molecules (the soldiers) to return to their original alignment after they have been stimulated by the magnetic field. (Liquids have long T1 times.) A T1 image shows good anatomical detail of the brain.
- *T2-weighted:* The rate at which magnetization is lost. A T2 image is best for showing contrast between types of tissues. It has less detail than a T1 image.

TABLE 2-2

CT and MRI: What's the Difference?

Computed Tomography	Magnetic Resonance Imaging
Easier to obtain	
Less expensive	
Scanning time 20 minutes	Scanning time up to an hour
Less sensitive	More sensitive
Shows bone and calcification well	Shows bone poorly
Uses x-rays	Does not use x-rays
Uses an iodine-based contrast agent	Contrast not iodine-based
Can be used for people with pacemakers or metallic implants	Cannot be used for people who have pacemakers or iron-based metallic implants
Shows skull base tumors poorly	Shows good detail of skull base tumors

Computed Tomography	Magnetic Resonance Imaging
Shows low-grade tumors poorly	Shows low-grade tumors well
Not good at showing swelling	Good at showing swelling

Positron Emission Tomography (PET)

Unlike CT and MRI, positron emission tomography (PET) gives us a view of the brain's metabolic activity—that is, the way in which it converts glucose into energy. To assess this conversion, the test measures levels of injected glucose (sugar) or methionine (amino acid) in the brain. This is a useful test in revealing brain tumors that rapidly metabolize, that is, use up a lot of energy from the glucose or methionine; these tumors include malignant gliomas or metastases. A PET scan is generally not used to diagnose brain tumors, but it can give your doctor additional information about your tumor.

PET scanning may help to determine the difference between a benign and a malignant tumor because malignant tumors are more metabolically active than benign tumors. It can also show the effects of treatment—from radiation, chemotherapy, or steroid medications—on the tumor; it can help to distinguish dead tissue resulting from radiation therapy from a recurrent tumor; it can demonstrate which parts of a tumor are most metabolically active; and it may help physicians detect recurrent brain tumors.

The downside of a PET scan is that it can have both false-positive and false-negative results; it is expensive and not fully covered by many insurance companies; it may not be available in all centers; and it shows little anatomical detail. A recent method of combining PET and CT has helped us to correlate PET results with the anatomical details shown on a CT scan.

How Does It Work? A PET scan requires a mildly radioactive substance (such as fluoro-deoxy-glucose, or FDG) to be injected into a vein in your arm. About 40 minutes after this injection, images are taken; often these images are combined with a CT scan, which takes about 30 minutes. Once inside the brain, the radioactive substance produces gamma rays. The PET scanner measures the energy given off by these rays, and its computer uses these measurements to create images in sections, much like regular CT images. Tumor cells, which crave sugar, take in more of the radioactive substance than normal cells, so they look brighter than healthy cells on the PET scan.

How Soon Will I Know the Results? A nuclear medicine radiologist will have the results of your PET scan in three or four days.

Single-Photon Emission Computed Tomography (SPECT)

Like PET, single-photon emission computed tomography (SPECT) uses radioisotopes to show the metabolic changes in the brain. Also, like PET, it may help to distinguish dead tissue from tumor.

How Does It Work? Radiopharmaceuticals (isotopes like Technetium-99 or thallium-201 chloride) are given intravenously. These isotopes give off photons in the brain that are "photographed" by a rotating gamma camera. A computer then uses the images to create cross-sectional pictures of the brain. This takes approximately half an hour.

What Does It Feel Like? Aside from the injection of the radioactive substance, a SPECT scan is painless.

How Soon Will I Know the Results? Usually the results are available within 72 hours.

Angiography

Angiography shows the blood vessels—arteries, veins, and sinuses—in the brain. It can be done with either CT or MR imaging; with MR angiography or CT angiography, the scans are taken in a special way to emphasize the blood vessels, but to the patient they are just like the usual CT or MRI scans.

Angiography also may be done with injection of an iodine dye into the arteries. A catheter is inserted into the femoral artery in the groin and threaded up to the brain. This is an invasive procedure. X-ray films are taken to outline the vessels so that they show up clearly on the films. This kind of angiography is used if a tumor is thought to be vascular; that is, thought to have a rich blood supply. It may show clusters of blood vessels that are characteristic of a tumor. In some situations it may also be used to block blood vessels of the tumor by embolization (small particles are used to block blood flow). This procedure, done by specialists called endovascular neurosurgeons or interventional radiologists, is an important adjunct to surgery in some institutions.

What Does It Feel Like? Transfemoral angiography is sometimes uncomfortable and some patients experience a sensation of heat during the injection. Sedation is usually given for this test. Be sure to tell your health care team if you are allergic to shellfish, because the iodine in this dye can cause an unpleasant reaction.

How Long Will It Last? Transfemoral angiography may last several hours, as each vessel has to be identified and injected.

How Soon Will I Know the Results? The results from this test are often available in two days.

Other Tests

Diagnostic imaging scans can provide a great deal of information about the structure of your brain and some of its function. Other tests can help to assess the function of the brain more accurately, however. These include an electroencephalogram (EEG) and evoked responses, and tests of vision and hearing. The lumbar puncture is also used sometimes in brain tumor diagnosis.

Electroencephalography (EEG) and Evoked Responses

Like powerful computers, our brains are abuzz with electrical activity. One way to record this activity is through an electroencephalogram (EEG). An EEG can detect seizure activity, areas of abnormal electrical activity, and the absence of electrical activity. If a tumor is present, it may show slow activity because the tumor blocks normal brain waves or it may show "spikes" that suggest brain irritability caused by the tumor.

Evoked responses are EEG responses to a particular stimulus; these provide information about the function of important parts of the brain. The three common evoked responses are:

1. *The visual evoked response (VER).* This test measures the time it takes for an electrical impulse to travel from the retina (in the eye) to the occipital lobe after a visual stimulus. The stimulus is usually a shifting visual pattern like a checkerboard or lines.
2. *The brain stem auditory evoked response (BAER).* The BAER tests the hearing pathways from the ear to the temporal lobe. The stimulus is a clicking noise.
3. *The somatosensory evoked response (SSER).* This test assesses sensory pathways from the skin to the cortex in the brain. The stimulus is usually given to the leg or the hand.

How Does It Work? An EEG measures electrical activity in the brain. Evoked responses measure electrical activity that mirrors a stimulus such as touch, vision, or sound. If a tumor is present, the activity is slowed because of the blockage caused by the tumor.

What Does It Feel Like? Get ready for a bad hair day! On the morning of your EEG, don't put gel or spray on your hair. The EEG technician will need to attach electrode leads to your head with a clear sticky glue, and some hair products can interfere with the gel's ability to stick. If your hair is thick, the technician may need to shave small areas in order to make a place to attach the electrodes.

How Long Will It Last? An EEG can last from 20 minutes to about 2 hours. In some instances, patients need to stay in the hospital for a whole week while an EEG monitors their brain waves.

How Soon Will I Know the Results? An *epileptologist,* a neurologist with special training in epilepsy and reading EEG results, will analyze your EEG. This may take up to a week.

Visual Field Tests (Perimetry)

Perimetry is used to test for complete or partial loss of the visual field, the whole area of our vision. Some tumors press on visual pathways and lead to loss of vision in part of the field.

How Does It Work? A neuro-ophthalmologist, an eye doctor with expertise in areas of the nervous system that relate to the eye, usually performs this test.

What Does It Feel Like? Visual field tests are not painful. In fact, they're just like a regular eye exam in which you tell the eye doctor whether you can see objects in the periphery of your vision.

How Long Will It Last? Visual field tests generally last 20 to 30 minutes.

How Soon Will I Know the Results? The results of visual field tests are available immediately. The neuro-ophthalmologist will explain them to you and will send them to your neurosurgeon.

Audiometry (Hearing Tests)

Hearing tests are used to assess your hearing and to tell whether your hearing difficulty comes from a bone (conduction) problem or nerve damage (sensorineural loss). Sensorineural loss, which is caused by pressure on the cochlear nerve or other damage to it, may involve a vestibular schwannoma, a type of benign tumor.

How Does It Work? A hearing specialist (an audiologist) usually performs this test; it simply involves listening to tones or other sounds.

What Does It Feel Like? It is completely pain-free.

How Long Will It Last? Usually about half an hour.

How Soon Will I Know the Results? The audiologist knows the test results right away, but he or she may wish to have further interpretation from an ear, nose, and throat (ENT) doctor, neurologist, or neurosurgeon.

Lumbar Puncture (Spinal Tap)

A lumbar puncture is a test used to obtain cerebrospinal fluid for analysis. It involves placement of a very fine needle into the lower back.

How Does It Work? In a lumbar puncture, a very fine needle samples cerebrospinal fluid. For this test, you will lie in a curled-up position and your lower back will be numbed with novocaine.

What Does It Feel Like? The first thing you will feel is the wetness of the prep solution, then the doctor pressing on your back. You may then feel a slight sting during the injection of lidocaine and perhaps some pressure. If the needle is close to a nerve, you may also feel some temporary burning, numbness, or tingling in one leg. Occasionally, the test can be quite painful if the nerves are stuck together or irritated by the needle for some other reason.

How Long Will It Last? The entire procedure lasts about 20 minutes. When it's over, rest for up to an hour before you go home. Lie flat while your body builds up the fluid again in your system, to make up for the fluid that was removed for the sample. When you sit up after this resting period, you may experience a spinal headache (forehead and neck pain), so have someone available to drive you home. Don't go to the gym or plan to do much for about 24 hours.

How Soon Will I Know the Results? The spinal fluid pressure is known immediately; other results of a spinal tap are usually available in one week.

You have had diagnostic tests to determine if you have a tumor and learned what type of tumor it is. In Part Two, you will learn how physicians classify brain tumors and find pertinent information about the type of tumor that concerns you.

PART TWO

■

Types of
Brain Tumors

For many years now at our hospital, our nurses and social workers have run a brain tumor support group for patients and their families. Recently, I was asked to address the group. Sitting with them, I realized how each patient's tumor was different from that of the others' in the room.

Arlene was an impeccably dressed fifty-five-year-old woman. She had just had surgery to remove a *meningioma*, the most common type of benign brain tumor. The good news about meningiomas is that when we diagnose them early, as in Arlene's case, we can remove them surgically before they do significant permanent damage to the brain. Arlene was learning to cope with the fact that she would now be considered a tumor "survivor."

Shirley was sitting across from her. Shirley also had a meningioma, but she was not as lucky as Arlene. Her tumor had wrapped itself around the base of her brain, ensnaring blood vessels as well as the nerves of hearing and facial movement. She had gone into surgery with double vision and hearing loss. She came out with the same double vision and slightly worse hearing loss. Shirley was trying to deal with the future implications of these problems and the likelihood of needing further treatment such as radiation for the tumor that was left.

Across the way from her was Charles. He looked like a movie star, although he had just had surgery two weeks ago. If you looked behind his right ear you could see a small incision. He tended to turn his head to the left when he was trying to hear. He would explain to those who wished to listen that he had had a vestibular schwannoma, a brain tumor that stems from the eighth cranial nerve, and that he had done very well except for hearing loss that had not been improved by surgery.

Carolyn sat beside him. She was twenty-eight years old and had a sudden seizure after the birth of her first baby. After some tests, her physician discovered that she had a *glioma*, a common type of brain tumor that arises from the brain tissue itself. Although Carolyn's tumor was low-grade—that is, slow growing—and she had it removed, she was still terrified about its effect on her and her family.

Charlotte had a very broad nose and a large jaw and hands that looked more like spades than hands. I recognized immediately, just by looking at her, that she most likely had a condition called acromegaly, from a benign tumor on her pituitary gland. This condition has a characteristic pattern—in it the jaw juts out, the nose and cheekbones enlarge, and the soft tissues of the body get very thick.

Another striking person was James. He had a small head and small stature overall. He was mentally slower than many others in the group, and while he declared himself a ten-year survivor of a highly malignant pediatric brain tumor called *medulloblastoma*, now he is faced with the after-effects of his treatment.

Charmaine was sitting in the corner. She, too, had a distinctive physical appearance. Her face was bloated and her body was obese. Her hair was sparse and she had multiple bruises on her arms. Most of these changes were from the steroid medications we use to treat a serious malignant tumor called *glioblastoma*.

Ralph and Jennifer sat at the back of the room. They both suffered from *metastatic brain tumors*. Ralph had surgery for lung cancer last year. He was attending this support group because the lung cancer had spread to his brain, and he was trying to decide whether to have surgery or radiation. Jennifer's story was similar, except that her metastatic brain tumor had developed six years after her breast cancer was diagnosed. She had the same kind of tough decision to make as her friend.

Primary and Secondary Brain Tumors

The support group provided a poignant example of the variable nature of brain tumors. Although more than 100 different types of brain tumors exist, nine of ten brain tumors are of the types experienced by the members of this group. These brain tumors fall into two broad categories: *primary brain tumors,* those that originate in the brain, and *secondary (or metastatic) brain tumors,* which develop when cancer cells from elsewhere in the body travel to the brain.

> For all brain tumors, definitive diagnosis can only be made by surgery with pathological examination of tissue. MRI or CT scans or other images may suggest the tumor type, but they are not definitive.

We can also divide primary brain tumors (the tumors that originate in the brain) into those that are *benign* (nonspreading) and those that are *malignant,* or likely to spread.

The following table summarizes these tumor types, and a complete listing is found in the appendix.

Tumors Originating in the Brain (Primary Brain Tumors)

Generally benign tumors	Malignant tumors and tumors with uncertain behavior
	Gliomas
Meningiomas	Astroglial neoplasms
Pituitary adenomas	Astrocytomas
Vestibular schwannomas	Anaplastic astrocytomas
Craniopharyngiomas	Glioblastomas
Pilocytic astrocytomas	Oligodendroglial neoplasms
	Oligodendrogliomas
Colloid cysts	Anaplastic oligodendrogliomas
Hemangioblastomas	Mixed gliomas
Epidermoid cysts	Gangliogliomas
	Ependymomas
	Lymphomas
	Medulloblastomas

Generally benign tumors	Malignant tumors and tumors with uncertain behavior
	Germ-cell tumors
	Pineoblastomas and pineocytomas
	Chordomas and chondrosarcomas
	Choroid-plexus carcinomas

The brain tumors that are secondary to cancer elsewhere in the body (metastatic brain tumors) can also be divided into two categories: single or multiple metastases in the brain; and meningeal carcinomatosis, or cancer that is metastatic to the cerebral meninges, the sheets of tissue that surround the brain. Meningeal carcinomatosis represents approximately 5 percent of all metastatic brain tumors; breast, lung, and melanoma are the most common primary tumors that produce this problem.

How Do Doctors Classify Brain Tumors?

In addition to the diagnosis of a tumor type, you may also hear a tumor referred to by cell type and grade. As I mentioned in chapter 1, tumors that originate in various cells in the brain (such as astrocytes, oligoden-drocytes, and schwann cells) take the names of those cells; for example, astrocytomas, oligodendrogliomas, and schwannomas.

Pathologists (specialists who read biopsy samples) who evaluate brain tumors may also assign tumors such as meningiomas and gliomas a grade that refers to their *histologic* appearance—that is, the way their cells look under a microscope. They are particularly interested in whether cells show signs of malignancy or aggressive behavior. Most health institutions use the World Health Organization (WHO) system for grading gliomas, with grade I (low grade) referring to tumors that appear least likely to spread and grade IV (high grade) referring to tumors that appear to be most malignant. The WHO classification is given in detail in the appendix. Pathologists grade tumors according to the highest grade of cell that they see in a biopsy specimen.

Keep in mind as you hear these numbers that diagnostic labels are not set in stone. Your tumor grade may change, for instance, if the tumor grows. Tumor grades may increase; they usually don't decrease, even after

treatment. There also may be variations in the way differen[t]
view the tissue samples that they see—and often they see [a]
part of the tumor. For now, these numbers will help your hea[lth]
decide on which treatment is best for you.

In addition to these tumor classifications, your physician may assign a *Karnofsky performance score (KPS)* ranging from 0 to 100 (100 being normal function), according to your ability to perform daily tasks.

Bigger May Be Better

The size of a brain tumor may not matter nearly as much as where it's located. You may have a very large tumor that is benign and can be taken out readily, or you may have a very small tumor that is much more difficult to deal with because it is pressing on a delicate area such as your optic nerve, the nerve in your brain that affects your vision.

In the following chapters, we will describe various types of brain tumors and summarize their treatment. It is important to understand, however, that these are only general guidelines for treatment. Usually, specific treatment decisions are made by a hospital brain tumor board that includes surgeons, radiation oncologists, oncologists, radiologists, and neuropathologists.

In this part, the first three chapters cover primary brain tumors and the fourth chapter provides information about metastatic brain tumors. To begin, in chapter 3, I will describe three of the most common primary brain tumors: meningiomas, pituitary adenomas, and vestibular schwannomas.

3

———■———

Meningiomas, Pituitary Adenomas, and Vestibular Schwannomas

The doctor said I had a meningioma on my cerebellum. That didn't sound too bad until he said it was a brain tumor.
— Beau Dyer, patient with a brain tumor

Meningiomas

Susan, an extremely accomplished fifty-five-year-old woman, was CEO of her own business. She was leading a meeting one day when her arm became slightly numb. At first she thought she was having a stroke, but the numbness went away almost immediately.

Her primary care doctor was concerned that she may have had a mini-stroke—a transient ischemic attack, or TIA—and sent Susan to the radiology department of the hospital for a scan called MR angiography. (You may remember from the last chapter that this test reveals how blood is flowing through the brain's blood vessels.) The scan showed that Susan's arteries were fine, but it revealed a large menigioma, a tumor that is located in the lining of the brain. Susan was referred to a neurosurgeon, who suggested that the tumor could definitely be the origin of her numbness and that what she had experienced was probably a very mild seizure. She now had to decide whether to have the tumor removed or to take anticonvulsant medications and watch and wait.

Any one of us could be Susan. If you have just been diagnosed with a meningioma, you're not alone: meningiomas are among the most common brain tumors. In fact, they constitute about one-quarter of all primary brain tumors—tumors that originate in the brain. Most often these slow-growing tumors occur in otherwise healthy women, like Susan, at midlife. They are twice as common in women as in men, and they rarely occur in children.

Many patients with meningiomas have lost part of chromosome 22, which contains a tumor-suppressor gene. As I mentioned in chapter 1, cells use these genes to divide during development, but then are turned off. If this does not happen, normal cells can continue to divide abnormally—they become tumor cells. Female hormones may affect the growth of meningiomas: they may enlarge during pregnancy, and are more common in people who have had breast cancer. These tumors also have been linked to a genetic disorder called neurofibromatosis and to previous radiation therapy to the brain.

Fortunately, nine in ten meningiomas are benign; they don't tend to spread outside of the brain. Malignant meningiomas can spread (metastasize) to the lung and other organs, but this is rare.

What Are Meningiomas?

Until now, you may never have heard of meningiomas. They are relatively common tumors, occurring in 95 people per 100,000. These tumors develop in the meninges, the lining of the brain. Usually they grow inward from these membranes and exert pressure on the brain or spinal cord. They can cause seizures or loss of brain function. Often they can be removed safely with surgery, but radiation may be a useful additional treatment.

Symptoms of a Meningioma

Meningiomas often show no symptoms. Because they tend to affect middle-aged women, when symptoms do occur they can be confused with other disorders that can occur in women in that age group: autoimmune and endocrine disorders, depression, or symptoms of menopause.

Possible symptoms of this tumor include:

- Seizures
- Headaches
- Weakness or loss of sensation in an arm or leg
- Confusion

- Diminished vision or double vision
- Hearing loss
- Personality changes

These symptoms of meningioma depend on the tumor's location. Meningiomas on surface areas of the brain (*convexity meningiomas*) may cause seizures or a gradually increasing problem with muscular weakness or partial paralysis on one side of the body (*hemiparesis*); sensory problems like numbness, tingling or burning, or a lost sense of smell; lack of coordination; or a change in personality.

Parasagittal tumors, that is, tumors that arise between the two hemispheres of the brain, may cause confusion, headaches, seizures, or weakness in one or both legs.

Subfrontal and *sphenoid ridge tumors* are often surprisingly large before they cause symptoms. Like *parasellar meningiomas,* they develop behind the eye and can produce visual symptoms.

Other less common meningiomas include *optic nerve sheath meningiomas,* which may cause blindness in one eye; *cerebellopontine angle meningiomas,* which may cause hearing loss and facial numbness; and *spinal cord meningiomas,* which can lead to numbness or tingling in arms or legs. *Tentorial notch* and *intraventricular meningiomas* may occur with almost no symptoms. Double vision (*diplopia*) may occur with meningiomas of the cavernous sinus or those that compress the sixth cranial nerve.

Diagnosis of a Meningioma

A CT or MRI scan with contrast enhancement is an excellent test to diagnose a meningioma. If a meningioma is found, the tumor is usually an enhancing mass with a sharp margin, and it comes from the lining of the brain. In some cases, a biopsy is needed for certain diagnosis, but this is one tumor that is quite characteristic on an MRI because it is based in the dura of the brain and has a smooth border.

Meningiomas are graded in this way:

1. Grade I (benign meningiomas) are slow-growing, localized tumors, with defined borders. Ninety percent of meningiomas are grade I.
2. Grade II (also called atypical meningiomas) grow more quickly and may spread into the surrounding brain lining. Once removed

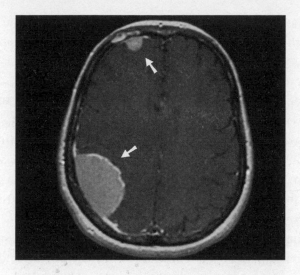

**Figure 3-1.   An MRI scan of two meningiomas
arising from the lining of the brain.**

The smaller one (top) is in the right frontal region (remember that right is on the left of the scan) and the larger one (bottom) is in the right parietal region. These tumors come from the meninges and compress brain tissue.

surgically, they may recur. Five to ten percent of meningiomas are atypical.

3. Grade III (also called malignant or anaplastic meningiomas) are aggressive tumors and compose about 1 percent of all meningiomas.

Treatment of Meningiomas

We usually consider four treatment options for meningiomas:

1. *Observation.* For older adults and for people with small meningiomas that are not producing symptoms, observation may be the best approach. If this is the option that you and your doctor choose, you will need to have regular MRI or CT scans, at least every year. For more guidance on "watching and waiting," see chapter 10.

2. *Surgery.* Many people with a meningioma eventually have surgery. Meningiomas that are causing symptoms, as well as those that are enlarging

or causing swelling, should be removed surgically rather quickly. Young patients with meningiomas that are easy to reach surgically are also good candidates for this form of treatment, because without surgery the tumor is likely to grow over their lifetime.

Recent advances in technique and approaches to these tumors have made surgery increasingly safe. The use of image-guided surgery, surgery with an operating microscope, and an increasing commitment to the safest possible surgery have made surgery for meningiomas much less risky than in the past. The risk of removing the meningioma depends on its relationship to surrounding tissue, including the brain tissue, blood vessels, and nerves.

If your health-care team recommends surgery, look for a surgical center that has sophisticated brain-monitoring equipment and operating microscopes. Meningiomas such as intraventricular meningiomas (that is, tumors within the brain's ventricles), pineal region meningiomas, skull base meningiomas, and suprasellar tumors require special expertise.

3. *Radiation.* For invasive or enlarging tumors in areas that are difficult to remove surgically, focused radiation can be a successful alternative. Radiation also may be used after surgery to prevent any remaining cells from spreading or to treat recurrence. I discuss the types of radiation in chapter 12.

4. *Chemotherapy.* In addition to watchful waiting, surgery, and radiation, we are trying chemotherapy for very aggressive meningiomas. The drugs include cyclophosphamide, adriamycin, and vincristine (CAV); dacarbazine and adriamycin; and high-dose ifosfamide. Some recent studies suggest that mifepristone, hydroxyurea, and interferon alfa-2b (IFNa-2b) may be helpful for malignant meningiomas. However, these therapies do not appear to be very effective. For more information about chemotherapy drugs, see chapter 13.

Follow-up Care

We recommend regular follow-up MRI or CT scans at one- to three-year intervals for patients who have had a meningioma. Tumor recurrence after surgery is more common for atypical and malignant meningiomas than for typical meningiomas. Additional surgery, stereotactic radiosurgery, or intensity-modulated radiotherapy may be used for recurrence

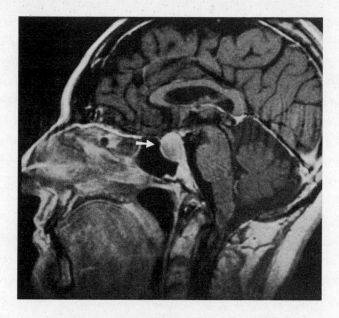

**Figure 3-2.   A sideways—sagittal—view of a
pituitary adenoma on an MRI scan.**

The arrow points to the adenoma, which enlarges the sella turcica and extends toward
the optic chiasm. This tumor is best removed by surgery going through the sphenoid
sinus. (Image courtesy of Dr. Liangge Hsu, Brigham and Women's Hospital)

(see chapters 11 and 12). These tumors are less likely than many other
brain tumors to lead to death.

Pituitary Adenomas

Robert, an active twenty-eight-year-old attorney, could not understand why his shoes and gloves seemed to get smaller each year. He
also noticed that his jaw appeared to be enlarging, although he didn't
think this was possible in a full-grown man. One night, a guest at a
party asked him whether he had ever had pituitary surgery. This
turned into a discussion about a disease called acromegaly, which the
fellow guest had diagnosed from across the room by the appearance
of Robert's face. Robert saw a physician and got an MRI, which
showed a pituitary tumor. The tumor was removed and he has been
fine ever since, although his face and hands have not completely
returned to normal.

Acromegaly is one of the diseases that can be caused by a pituitary adenoma. Pituitary adenomas, which account for about 10 percent of all brain tumors, develop in the pituitary gland. This gland is located at the base of the brain and controls the body's growth and metabolism through the release of chemical messengers called hormones.

Most pituitary tumors are benign, slow-growing masses that arise in a part of the pituitary gland called the *adenohypophysis*. Small (less than 10 millimeters) pituitary adenomas are called *microadenomas;* larger ones are called *macroadenomas*.

Symptoms of Pituitary Adenomas

The symptoms of pituitary adenomas fall into two general categories: those created by *endocrine syndromes,* caused by tumors that secrete too much or too little of a given hormone, and those created by syndromes of *mass effect,* caused by non-secreting tumors that create problems by pushing on important structures in the brain.

Endocrine syndromes may reflect increased or decreased production of certain hormones. The following syndromes are associated with increased pituitary function:

1. The most common endocrine syndrome is related to a pituitary tumor called a *prolactinoma*. This tumor secretes too much prolactin, the hormone linked to milk production. In premenopausal women, a prolactinoma may cause periods to stop (*amenorrhea*) and milk to flow from the breasts (*galactorrhea*). In men, it can cause headache, loss of vision, impotence, and, rarely, galactorrhea.

2. *Acromegaly,* a disorder caused by excessive secretion of growth hormone from the pituitary gland, is characterized by gigantism (excessive growth) in children and adolescents and by a broad chin and nose, prominent forehead, gap teeth, and wide bones in the fingers and toes in adults. More important than these skeletal changes, acromegaly can cause metabolic abnormalities such as disease of the heart muscle (*cardiomyopathy*) and diabetes mellitus.

3. Too much secretion of a hormone called ACTH leads to *Cushing's disease.* This unpleasant disease leads to obesity, stripes on the skin, fragile

capillary blood vessels, and—in women—an abnormal collection of fatty tissue in the area where you would pat yourself on the upper back. Cushing's disease may also cause diabetes mellitus, osteoporosis, and depression.

4. People who have had one or both adrenal glands removed surgically can develop *Nelson's syndrome,* a disorder caused by overproduction of adrenocorticotropic hormone (ACTH). This syndrome is characterized by abnormally dark skin (hyperpigmentation) and a pituitary tumor that tends to be very aggressive.

5. Some rare tumors secrete too much thyroid hormone.

Mass effect. The most common type of pituitary adenoma a surgeon sees is a silent or "non-functioning" pituitary adenoma. This tumor does not secrete functioning hormones, although sometimes it can produce fragments of hormones called the alpha subunit. Symptoms of mass effect include:

- *Headache.* Often felt at the top of the head, with no particular distinguishing characteristics.
- *Visual field loss.* If the tumor is pressing on the optic nerve, the person may experience vision loss on one or both sides.
- *Headache, nausea, vomiting,* and *drowsiness.* Occur if the tumor is compressing the third ventricle of the brain.
- In *hypopituitarism,* the pituitary gland functions less well and secretes too few hormones. People with this syndrome tend to be overweight with soft pale skin and low energy. They may lose facial and body hair.
- About 1 percent of patients with a pituitary tumor will experience *pituitary apoplexy*—a pituitary stroke. This may cause severe headache, nausea, vomiting, confusion, dulled reflexes, and difficulty with sight.

Diagnosis of a Pituitary Adenoma
We do several types of tests—radiological scans, blood tests, and eye exams—to evaluate a pituitary adenoma. You may meet endocrinologists, ophthalmologists, and neurosurgeons in this evaluation.

1. *Imaging.* An MRI is the best imaging test to detect a pituitary adenoma. This type of scan will reveal small tumors within the gland and the full extent of larger tumors. It will show the tumor's relation to the skull and brain stem, as well as its relation to the *optic chiasm,* the structure where the fibers of the optic nerves cross.

A CT scan may show a large pituitary tumor, but detail on this scan is obscured by bone. It is not unusual for CT scans to miss a pituitary adenoma.

2. *Blood tests.* If your doctor suspects that you have a pituitary tumor, he or she will have you undergo some blood tests to find out what is happening with your hormone levels. These endocrine tests may include baseline prolactin, growth hormone, and 8 A.M. (fasting) cortisol levels, as well as thyroid function tests. These tests may show elevations of the hormone that suggest a tumor. If these levels are normal, it may be worthwhile to have your luteinizing hormone (LH), follicle-stimulating hormone (FSH), and alpha subunit levels tested also; these are less common hormones that may be elevated in tumors.

- *Your prolactin level:* A level above 20 ng/ml (nanograms/milliliter, the unit of measurement for prolactin) is abnormal, but this level is sometimes elevated without a tumor. A prolactin-producing tumor is almost certainly present if the level is above 200 ng/ml.
- *Your growth hormone level:* A baseline (fasting) growth hormone level greater that 10 ng/ml indicates an excessive amount of growth hormone; the usual cause is a pituitary tumor. Measurements of IGF-1 (insulin growth factor) may also be useful in making this diagnosis.
- *Your ACTH level:* To determine whether a pituitary adenoma is producing too much of the hormone ACTH, two tests are used: first, high (fasting) cortisol or 24-hour urinary corticosteroids; second, documenting that this high level is not suppressed when you are given a drug called dexamethasone by mouth. Sometimes ACTH is also measured in the petrosal sinus, a vein just beside the pituitary gland.

3. *Eye tests.* An eye specialist who performs a visual field test may detect an effect of these tumors on vision.

Treatment of a Pituitary Adenoma

Once your diagnosis is clear, your treatment options will depend on the type of pituitary tumor you have.

1. *Drug therapy.* For *prolactinomas,* the preferred initial treatment is bromocriptine or cabergoline, drugs that shrink the tumor and decrease the secretion of prolactin. These are expensive but effective pills; side effects include stomach upset, nausea, eye irritation, and low blood pressure. Your health-care team may prescribe a medication called octreotide (Sandostatin) if you have an adenoma that produces growth hormone. This is given by injection, but long-acting forms are being produced now.

2. *Surgery.* For non-functioning adenomas that produce growth hormone and for Cushing's disease, surgery to remove the tumor is usually effective. Surgery also may be helpful for patients with a prolactinoma who want to get pregnant or if there is rapid visual loss from any kind of tumor. This surgery is usually done through the nose and the sphenoid sinus— called a *transsphenoidal operation.* This can be done with an endoscope or an operating microscope. If the tumor is very large, the operation may involve opening the skull via a procedure called a craniotomy (see chapter 11).

3. *Radiation therapy.* Your doctor may recommend radiation therapy for a pituitary tumor that is not responding to drugs, that has recurred after surgery, or has not been removed completely through surgery. Chapter 12 describes the types and uses of radiation therapy.

Regardless of the therapy that you choose to destroy a pituitary tumor, your health-care team may continue to monitor you for many years with imaging, blood tests, and eye tests (visual field monitoring).

Vestibular Schwannomas (Acoustic Neuromas)

James was a thirty-four-year-old singer who was having increasing trouble hearing from his left ear. He went to his primary care doctor, who thought that this problem was probably early loss of bone conduction. She recommended that they continue to monitor his situation. However, as James's hearing steadily worsened over the

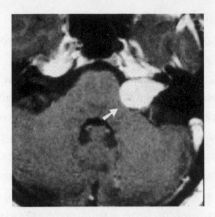

**Figure 3-3. A cross-section view of a
vestibular schwannoma on an MRI scan.**

The tumor presses on the brain stem and extends into the internal auditory meatus.

next few months, he began to ask for further testing. A hearing test called an *audiogram* showed that the problem was not in the ear itself, but rather related to the cochlear nerve—a sensorineural hearing loss.

The audiologist who performed the test recommended that James have an MRI scan. However, his primary care doctor said that this form of diagnostic testing was probably unnecessary and too expensive; instead, she asked James to see an ear, nose, and throat doctor (an ENT specialist, or otolaryngologist). The ENT specialist confirmed that James really should have an MRI scan. It revealed a 2-centimeter tumor on his vestibular nerve. He now had to decide what to do.

Vestibular schwannomas, which are also called acoustic neuromas, acoustic neurinomas, or acoustic or vestibular neurilemmomas, are benign tumors that arise from the vestibular portion of the eighth cranial nerve. They develop from Schwann cells, which produce myelin, the substance that coats and protects nerves. Vestibular schwannomas constitute less than 5 percent of all brain tumors. These slow-growing tumors generally occur in adults at midlife. People with a disorder called *neurofibromatosis type 2* (NF2) have a greater tendency to have these tumors.

Symptoms of a Vestibular Schwannoma

Vestibular schwannomas can cause a variety of symptoms:

- *Hearing loss* is the most common problem, but a person with a vestibular schwannoma may dismiss this hearing trouble for many years and attribute it to trauma or aging. These tumors almost always affect hearing on just one side, and they don't tend to affect one side more often than the other. The degree of hearing loss does not correspond to the size of the tumor. The hearing loss may be accompanied by a sensation of noise or ringing in the ear (tinnitus).
- *Vertigo* (dizziness) often accompanies these tumors.
- *Facial tingling, numbness (paresthesias),* or *paralysis* and *sensory loss* are sometimes related to a large tumor pressing on the trigeminal nerves.
- With increasing tumor size, *unsteadiness of gait or limb* and symptoms of increased fluid in the brain (*hydrocephalus*), including *headache* and *difficulty with balance and walking,* may occur.
- Large vestibular schwannomas that affect the lower cranial nerves can also cause *difficulty in swallowing and speaking.*

Diagnosis of a Vestibular Schwannoma

Most people who have a vestibular schwannoma first seek medical help because of difficulty hearing. Hearing can be tested by voice, by a tuning fork, or by an audiogram. The "brain stem-evoked response" adds further information.

If the results of your audiogram show sensorineural loss, your doctor will probably recommend that you have an MRI scan. This is the best type of imaging to view a vestibular schwannoma because it can even detect very small tumors if the test is given with a contrast (dye) called gadolinium. A CT of the internal auditory canal also may be useful to show widening of the canal caused by the tumor growing within it. For more information about these diagnostic tests, see chapter 2.

Treatment of a Vestibular Schwannoma

Depending on the size of the tumor and your symptoms, you may choose to watch and wait, have surgery to remove the tumor, or undergo radiation therapy. People with a vestibular schwannoma generally do not take chemotherapy.

1. *Observation.* If your tumor is not causing severe symptoms, it is less than 2 centimeters, and it is growing very slowly or not at all, one option is just to have an MRI scan every 6 to 12 months. If you have other major health problems, such as a heart condition, and your tumor is not getting bigger, waiting might be a good idea, even if the tumor is larger than 2 cm.

2. *Surgery.* Most patients with large or symptomatic vestibular schwannomas will need surgery. During an operation to remove this type of tumor, an otolaryngologist (ENT) is often an assisant surgeon with the neurosurgeon. If you choose to have this type of surgery, look for a surgical team that has experience with this procedure.

The nerves in the brain (the cranial nerves) are fragile. During surgery, if the vestibular schwannoma peels away from the facial and cochlear nerves easily, you will have a better outcome with fewer side effects. However, if the tumor is "sticky," so that it is more difficult to remove, the nerve may be jarred and there may be more long-term problems after surgery.

With today's neurosurgical techniques, we can monitor the cranial nerves during the operation so that we can remove vestibular schwannomas safely while sparing the function of the facial nerve. Sometimes we can preserve hearing as well, especially if we detect the tumor early. Sometimes we opt for incomplete removal of the tumor in order to spare the cochlear and facial nerves (and preserve hearing and prevent facial weakness); this means that the tumor may come back.

The good news is that once these tumors are completely removed, they usually don't recur. The less positive news is that there are several complications of surgery to remove a vestibular schwannoma. They include:

- *Hearing loss that may be lasting.* Although the risk for hearing loss remains, new techniques to monitor the auditory nerve during surgery are helping surgeons to preserve hearing function in many patients.
- *Facial weakness.* Surgeons today are able to monitor the facial nerve during surgery, so patients are experiencing less damage to this nerve. After surgery, some people who do experience facial weakness improve with special exercises and others just need time before their facial tone returns. Other people find they have difficulty eating for a while. For severe facial weakness, we can take a bit of another cranial

nerve and implant it to give the facial nerve a boost (this is called *reinervation*). If weak facial muscles make it difficult or impossible to close an eye, you may be at risk for an irritated cornea (abrasion). This problem is usually temporary, but if it persists, neurosurgeons, oculoplastic surgeons, or facial reconstructive surgeons can help with various procedures, including the implantation of a gold weight in your eyelid to protect your eye from too much exposure.

· *Dizziness, loss of balance (vestibular disturbances).*
· *Headaches.*
· *Cerebrospinal fluid leaks.* These leaks are usually treated by lowering the spinal fluid pressure with a lumbar drain or reoperating to seal the leak.

3. *Radiation therapy.* We often remove vestibular schwannomas surgically, but new radiation techniques have considerably changed their treatment. Some patients opt for focused radiation to control the growth of their tumors if they are concerned about facial weakness after surgery.

For individuals with small (less than 3 centimeters) vestibular schwannomas or for those with growing tumors who cannot undergo surgery, *stereotactic radiosurgery* may be a good option. This technique can be done with a gamma-emitting Co60 unit (the gamma knife), or a linear accelerator (the Novalis or other systems). It spares the brain tissue surrounding the tumor by making use of several convergent beams of radiation to deliver one high dose to the mass itself.

Similar techniques are *intensity-modulated radiation therapy* and *fractionated stereotactic radiotherapy,* which deliver focused doses of radiation in a number of treatment sessions. These are useful for larger tumors. For detailed information about these forms of radiation treatment, see chapter 12.

Meningiomas, pituitary adenomas, and vestibular schwannomas make up about 40 percent of primary brain tumors. They are generally benign, although occasionally they may become more aggressive. They are treated by observation, surgery, or radiation, and their treatment is usually very successful. In the next chapter, I will describe the symptoms, diagnosis, and treatment of gliomas, primary brain tumors that are more difficult to treat satisfactorily.

4

Gliomas

Like meningiomas, pituitary adenomas, and vestibular schwannomas, gliomas are primary brain tumors—they form in the brain itself. Almost half of all brain tumors originating in the brain are gliomas.

Gliomas arise from the glial cells of the central nervous system. The three major types of gliomas correspond to the forms of these glial cells: astrocytomas develop from astrocytes; oligodendrogliomas develop from oligodendrocytes; and ependymomas develop from ependymal cells. Mixed gliomas are brain tumors that arise from a combination of different types of cells. A particularly interesting kind of glioma is the ganglioglioma, which contains both neurons (nerve cells) and glial cells.

Gliomas may be either benign (such as the pilocytic astrocytoma) or malignant. They are most often located above the tentorium, a dividing line between the top and bottom of the brain in the cerebral hemispheres. Less often, they develop in the brain stem. I will first tell you about the characteristics that many gliomas have in common, and then I will explain more about each type of glioma.

Low-grade gliomas usually occur in people younger than 40; they may be astrocytomas, oligodendrogliomas, gangliogliomas, or ependymomas. Seizures and headaches are usually their first symptoms. Malignant gliomas can occur at any time in a person's life, but the average age at diagnosis is 50. Most often we detect these tumors on CT or MRI scans, but we can only make a definitive diagnosis and grade the tumor with a tissue biopsy.

How Gliomas Are Graded

Grade I (pilocytic astrocytoma): These tumors most often occur in children.

Grade II (low-grade glioma): These tumors include astrocytomas, oligodendrogliomas, mixed gliomas, gangliogliomas, and ependymomas.

Grade III (anaplastic glioma): These aggressive gliomas may be called anaplastic astrocytomas, anaplastic oligodendrogliomas, or anaplastic ependymomas.

Grade IV (glioblastoma multiforme): These very aggressive tumors contain dead tissue as well as new blood vessels.

Malignant gliomas don't usually metastasize out of the nervous system. However, they are quite aggressive within the brain itself and they can be difficult to eradicate, especially in people older than 65 years. These tumors are best treated with surgical removal followed by radiation therapy and chemotherapy. For recurrent tumors, new therapies including targeted growth factor inhibitors may be best. All of these treatment options are described in greater detail in Part Four.

Now I will discuss the specific types of gliomas, starting with the less aggressive (low-grade) tumors.

Pilocytic Astrocytomas

A pilocytic astrocytoma, or juvenile pilocytic astrocytoma, is the most benign (grade I) type of astrocytoma. Pilocytic astrocytomas are slow-growing tumors that occur primarily in children and adolescents. They may appear in the hypothalamus or optic nerve, where they are often inoperable, or in the cerebellum, or cerebral hemisphere, where they can be cured.

Diagnosis of Pilocytic Astrocytomas

Symptoms of this tumor depend on its location. In the cerebellum, it can produce headache and unsteadiness; in the optic nerve (where it is called an optic glioma), vision loss; and in the hypothalamus, a striking syndrome of early puberty, weight loss, and hyperactivity.

A CT or MRI scan may reveal enlargement of the affected area of the brain (such as the optic nerve or hypothalamus). A definitive diagnosis of this type of tumor requires biopsy, although if the patient has a disorder called neurofibromatosis, the physician may choose to watch and wait rather than attempt a surgical biopsy.

Treatment of Pilocytic Astrocytomas

1. *Observation.* Many pilocytic astrocytomas cannot be removed surgically because of their location. If a tumor is not growing, observation may be a better option than surgery.

2. *Surgery.* Surgery may be performed either for biopsy or removal of the tumor. A cerebellar pilocytic astrocytoma may be cured with surgery because it does not invade the cerebellum. In the optic nerve or hypothalamus, biopsy is usually the best option.

3. *Radiation therapy.* Radiation therapy may be used for patients with inoperable tumors, such as those in the optic nerve.

4. *Chemotherapy.* Chemotherapy, usually with a drug called temozolamide, is being tried in some children with inoperable pilocytic astrocytomas.

Astrocytomas

Carolyn was extremely excited because at last she had become pregnant. She had just delivered her baby when she had an episode she does not remember at all. Her husband, who was with her, remembers this experience as being one of the most frightening times of his life. Although their baby was doing fine, shortly after he was born, Carolyn turned her head to the right, her eyes became glassy, and her body began to shake.

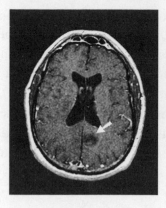 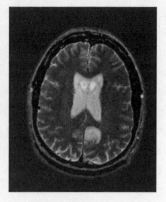

Figure 4-1.A.   **Figure 4-1.B.**

These "transaxial" views show the differences in MRI sequences. Figure 4-1.A is a T_1-weighted image with intravenous contrast. The tumor does not enhance and is seen as a dark sphere (arrow). Figure 4-1.B is a T_2-weighted image, with cerebrospinal fluid that shows up as white. This sequence is especially sensitive to water content or swelling. (Image courtesy of Dr. Liangge Hsu)

This lasted for approximately thirty seconds. Afterward, she could not be wakened for five minutes and then slowly she became herself again. She was sent to see a neurologist, who suggested that she should get an MRI scan. This scan revealed a dark area in the right frontal lobe of her brain which the radiologist thought was a low-grade astrocytoma.

Astrocytomas are so named because they are made up of astrocytes, star-shaped cells. These tumors can occur anywhere in the brain, but are rare in the cerebellum or brain stem.

Symptoms of Astrocytomas
Astrocytomas can cause headaches, difficulty in thinking, and seizures. Other symptoms may include vision problems, subtle personality changes, weakness on one side, or numbness.

Diagnosis of Astrocytomas
An MRI is generally the most reliable method for detecting astrocytomas because sometimes areas that appear normal on a CT scan are abnormal on an MRI. However, imaging is usually not enough for us to make a

definitive diagnosis because these tumors may resemble other tumors, multiple sclerosis, or brain inflammation. A biopsy is usually necessary.

Treatment of Astrocytomas

1. *Observation.* Sometimes a physician will recommend observation for what appears to be a low-grade astrocytoma. We tend to discourage this in our center because it is difficult to be sure that a tumor is low grade by MRI scanning alone.

2. *Surgery.* Surgery to remove as much of an astrocytoma as possible is usually the first step in treatment. Image-guided surgery with brain mapping (see chapter 11) has significantly improved management of these tumors, and the ability of surgeons to use MRI to view the tumor during surgery has been particularly important.

3. *Radiation.* In many centers, radiation may be recommended for astrocytomas that cannot be removed. A recent European study suggested that radiation does not prolong survival, but does delay time of recurrence.

Outcome of Astrocytomas

The major problem with astrocytomas is that with time they tend to progress to a more malignant grade. The survival time can vary from a few years to twenty or more. Long-term follow-up studies of astrocytomas that have been removed aggressively will help us to assess the prognosis of patients who undergo surgery to remove these tumors.

Anaplastic Astrocytomas

Anaplastic astrocytomas are similar to astrocytomas in appearance and in the constellation of symptoms. Usually a diagnosis can only be made with a biopsy. Anaplastic astrocytomas tend to be more aggressive than astrocytomas with a tendency to grow faster and to infiltrate the brain more extensively. They may result from progression of a low-grade astrocytoma. They are treated with radiation and chemotherapy. Patients with this tumor tend to survive from two to five years despite therapy.

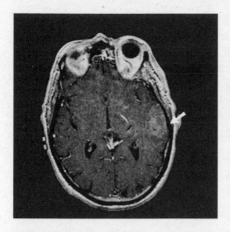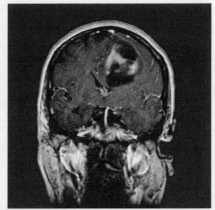

Figures 4-2.A and 4-2.B.   Anaplastic gliomas from two different patients.

Figure 4-2.A shows a left temporal anaplastic astrocytoma. It does not enhance and is a fairly subtle abnormality (arrow), but it is a malignant tumor. Figure 4-2.B shows a further advanced anaplastic astrocytoma in a coronal view. The white streaks represent new blood vessel formation in the tumor (angiogenesis). Anaplastic oligodendrogliomas have the same appearance as anaplastic astrocytomas.

Variants of anaplastic astrocytoma are:

• *Gemistocytic astrocytoma:* This type of tumor contains plump glial cells called gemistocytes. These tumors often recur.
• *Pleomorphic xanthoastrocytoma*: This type of Grade II–III tumor most often occurs in the temporal lobe of children and young adults.

Glioblastoma multiforme (Glioblastoma)

Charmaine was fifty-two years old when her behavior began to change in ways that she didn't recognize at first. She tended to fly off the handle more easily than in the past. When left alone, she was happy simply sitting by herself instead of being active. She tended to say things that she wouldn't have said four years ago. Her friends were not sure what this was all about and thought perhaps she was experiencing early senility. They finally convinced her to see a doctor, who recommended that she have a CT scan. After this imaging test, the technician asked her to stay until she could get a radiologist to take a look at the scan. It showed a large mass in the right side of her brain and she had a major brain operation to remove a glioblastoma shortly after that.

Glioblastomas develop in the cerebral hemispheres and spread quickly into the surrounding tissue of the brain. They occur in the prime of life; the median age of people in whom these tumors are diagnosed is 50 to 55 years.

Symptoms of a Glioblastoma

Headache, vomiting, nausea, and tiredness are all possible symptoms of a glioblastoma. As these tumors enlarge and put pressure on various structures of the brain, they can also cause seizures, weakness, or numbness on one side of the body, and problems with speech, vision, and memory.

Diagnosis of a Glioblastoma

On an enhanced MRI scan, this type of tumor appears to be necrotic in its center; that is, it may have a dark center that contains dead tissue. It may be surrounded by a white ring and swollen tissue. Without a tissue biopsy, however, it is sometimes difficult to determine whether a mass is a glioblastoma or an abscess, lymphoma, or metastatic tumor.

Treatment of a Glioblastoma

Glioblastomas spread extensively into the brain. Depending on where they are located, we can treat glioblastomas with surgery, stereotactic radiosurgery, radiation, chemotherapy, immunotherapy, or other new treatment options. I will describe these methods in detail in Part Four. No matter which therapy we choose, our goal is to relieve the pressure created by these tumors in the brain and to make the environment surrounding them unfavorable to their growth.

Oligodendrogliomas

Oligodendrogliomas (pronounced all-ih-go-dendro-gliomas) are gliomas that resemble clusters of oligodendrocytes, the cells that serve as insulators

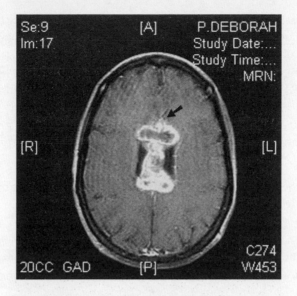

Figure 4-3.   MRI of a glioblastoma.

This is the most malignant type of primary brain tumor. Note the dark center, which suggests necrosis (dead tissue) (arrow) and the bright enhancement around it. (Image courtesy of Dr. Liangge Hsu)

for neurons. Under the microscope, oligodendrocytes are round cells that look like a fried egg with small blood vessels (capillaries) extending outward in a pattern that resembles chicken wire. These tumors often occur in young and middle-aged adults, and they sometimes occur in children. We detect them best with CT and MRI scans. To confirm the diagnosis, a biopsy is necessary.

Oligodendrogliomas are best treated by surgical removal of as much of the tumor as possible. In our experience, the best treatment for residual tumor is to observe it and then consider chemotherapy or radiation if it begins to grow. People with these tumors have a good overall prognosis.

Anaplastic Oligodendrogliomas

Joe, a very successful salesman, had just celebrated his forty-fifth birthday. He had generally been healthy, but one day he had trouble speaking. Although this difficulty was not severe, it was so different than his usual speech that he became worried and went to see his primary care physician. She set up an appointment for him to have a CT scan right away.

I saw him shortly after the CT was done; it revealed an enhancing mass in the left frontal area of his brain. It appeared to be close to the part of the brain that controls movement, but we felt it deserved an attempt at surgical removal. We removed 90 percent of the tumor, leaving a small amount deep in the white matter of the brain. He had no new deficits postoperatively.

His tumor turned out to be an anaplastic oligodendroglioma. With chemotherapy he is alive and well five years after surgery with no evidence of residual tumor.

Anaplastic oligodendrogliomas usually develop in adults at midlife. They appear to be resistant to radiation, but they may respond to chemotherapy.

Symptoms of an Anaplastic Oligodendroglioma
This tumor can cause headaches and seizures, or it may be asymptomatic.

Diagnosis of an Anaplastic Oligodendroglioma
Both CT and MRI scans can detect an anaplastic oligodendroglioma, but a biopsy is necessary to confirm the diagnosis.

Treatment of an Anaplastic Oligodendroglioma
Treatment options for people with this type of tumor include surgery, chemotherapy, and radiation. One of the most important recent developments in neuro-oncology has been the recognition that many of these tumors are sensitive to chemotherapy and that this can be predicted by a test of the tumor's chromosomes. Patients who have deletion of 1p19q chromosomes have a particularly good outcome. This is discussed further in chapter 13.

Mixed Gliomas

Mixed gliomas usually include both tumorous astrocytes and oligodendrocytes. They are generally treated the same as oligodendrogliomas.

Gangliogliomas

Gangliogliomas, tumors that contain both glial cells and neurons, can occur in people of all ages. In children, they are usually slow-growing lesions that do not tend to spread beyond their own borders. In adults, they may be more diffuse and occur in the cerebral hemispheres. They appear in men and women equally.

Symptoms of Gangliogliomas

Most people with a ganglioglioma first seek medical attention because of seizures. Other symptoms include headache; unsteadiness or lack of coordination when walking; muscular weakness or partial paralysis on one side of the body (*hemiparesis*); and a tingling or creeping sensation in the skin (*paresthesias*).

Diagnosis of Gangliogliomas

We can detect a ganglioglioma on either a CT or an MRI scan. On a CT scan, gangliogliomas frequently appear calcified and cystic. Biopsy specimens of these tumors show that they are composed of variable proportions of ganglion cells and glial cells. With the biopsy sample we can confirm the diagnosis of a ganglioglioma if the pathologist finds that both the neurons and glial cells have become tumorous.

Treatment of Gangliogliomas

1. *Observation.* In children with an apparent ganglioglioma in an area that would be difficult to reach surgically, observation is sometimes the best policy. However, a biopsy is usually necessary.

2. *Surgery.* The basic treatment for gangliogliomas and the best chance for a cure is complete removal of the tumor. If you have surgery to remove this type of tumor, afterward you will need to have annual MRIs to ensure that the tumor is gone.

3. *Radiation Therapy.* We recommend external beam radiation therapy (see chapter 12) if the tumor grows back after surgery or if we are not

able to remove the entire tumor. Sometimes we also advise this course of treatment if a biopsy shows that the ganglioglioma has anaplastic features; that is, if its cells have characteristics of a more aggressive tumor.

4. *Chemotherapy.* Some people have chemotherapy after surgery if a sample of the tumor indicates the tumor is malignant. It is generally the same chemotherapy as that used for malignant oligodendrogliomas.

Ependymomas

Ependymomas (pronounced eh-pen-di-momas) are rare; they make up less than 2 percent of all primary brain tumors. They occur primarily in young adults or children; one in ten brain tumors in children is an ependymoma. These tumors arise from the ependymal cells, which line the ventricles of the brain and the internal canal of the spinal cord. They can spread through the cerebrospinal fluid.

Symptoms of Ependymomas

These tumors can cause unsteadiness and symptoms associated with excessive fluid in the brain (*hydrocephalus*), including headache and swelling behind the eyes (*papilledema*).

Diagnosis of Ependymomas

A CT or MRI scan can detect this type of tumor, but as with other tumors, we can only confirm the diagnosis with a biopsy or surgical removal.

Treatment of Ependymomas

We treat ependymomas by removing as much as possible surgically, followed by radiation to both the brain and spinal cord to prevent the spread of tumor cells through the spinal column (called *intraspinal "drop" metastases*).

Now that you know how we manage gliomas, let's move on to chapter 5, where I will describe the other types of primary brain tumors that we see.

5

■

Other Primary Brain Tumors

In the last two chapters, I told you about some of the common primary brain tumors that we often see in our brain tumor clinic. In this chapter, you will find a guide to some unusual tumors that originate in the brain. These include benign tumors such as craniopharyngiomas, epidermoid and colloid cysts, choroid plexus papillomas, and hemangioblastomas, as well as malignant tumors: lymphomas, medulloblastomas, primitive neuroectodermal tumors, germ-cell tumors, pineal region tumors, chordomas, and choroid-plexus carcinomas.

Unusual Primary Benign Brain Tumors

Craniopharyngioma

A craniopharyngioma is a rare tumor that grows in the region of the optic nerves and hypothalmus. Although it is considered benign and we can remove it surgically, it can cause visual and endocrine problems because of its location. The hypothalamus is the part of the brain that regulates body temperature and hormones. It also affects hunger, thirst, moods, motivation, and sexual development.

This tumor is most commonly found in people between 10 and 30 years of age, but it can occur in individuals at either extreme of life. It grows from remnants of cells near the hypothalamus. Even though it is "benign," this tumor, because of its location, may act malignant as it recurs or continues to grow and compress the hypothalamus and the optic nerve.

Symptoms of a Craniopharyngioma

Craniopharyngiomas can crowd the pituitary gland, which is responsible for growth. In childhood or adolescence, these tumors can cause delayed puberty and other endocrine problems. Tish Reidy, a nurse at Children's Hospital in Boston, notes that these "funky tumors" can lead to diabetes insipidus, vision problems, sleep cycle problems, and learning disabilities in children.

In adults, craniopharyngiomas may cause sexual dysfunction, obesity, and visual loss. A patient may discover this type of tumor when he is feeling rundown and doesn't have enough energy to get out of bed in the morning. He or she may also have difficulty with eyesight and trouble reading.

Diagnosis of a Craniopharyngioma

Skull x-ray films may show that the *sella turcica,* a bone that surrounds the pituitary gland, is enlarged. These films may also show calcification.

The CT scan will show a rounded, often cystic mass and MRI may reveal multiple cystic areas.

Blood tests may uncover a variety of deficiencies in hormones from the pituitary gland; a specialist in hormone abnormalities—an endocrinologist—should become part of the treatment team.

Treatment of a Craniopharyngioma

1. *Observation.* If there are no symptoms and the tumor is small, observation may be appropriate.

2. *Surgery.* Most people with a craniopharyngioma have surgery to remove as much of the tumor as possible. As I will explain in more detail

in chapter 11, this can be done as a craniotomy (through the skull) or sometimes as a transsphenoidal procedure (through the nose).

3. *Radiation therapy.* An important adjunct to surgery for craniopharyngiomas, radiation therapy diminishes the likelihood that the tumor will recur.

After treatment, memory loss, changes in behavior and appetite, and endocrine dysfunction can occur. A person with this type of tumor may need to take hormone therapy to maintain a normal balance of hormones.

Epidermoid and Dermoid Cysts

Epidermoid cysts contain fragments of skin; dermoid cysts contain skin and other appendages such as hair follicles. These rare tumors are really just pieces of skin enclosed in the brain because of a mistake in fetal development.

Symptoms of Epidermoid and Dermoid Cysts
These cysts often do not cause symptoms, though they may lead to seizures, double vision, facial numbness, or symptoms of hydrocephalus.

Diagnosis of Epidermoid and Dermoid Cysts
The diagnosis is best made with special sequences of MRI scans that may distinguish these cysts from other cysts of the brain. The diagnosis can be made definitively by removal of the cyst.

Treatment of Epidermoid and Dermoid Cysts
The treatment for both dermoid and epidermoid tumors is surgery to remove as much of the cyst as possible. Usually not all can be removed, and the tumor may recur after many years. Further surgery can be done. However, because this type of mass develops slowly, it may not cause problems for many years.

Radiation therapy is not helpful in the treatment of these cysts.

Colloid Cysts

Colloid cysts are rare but curable lesions that occur almost exclusively in adults.

Symptoms of Colloid Cysts

These cysts develop in the third ventricle of the brain and can block the flow of cerebrospinal fluid (CSF). This blockage creates pressure that can cause headache, dizziness, and nausea.

Diagnosis of Colloid Cysts

We may use CT or MRI scans to diagnose these cysts.

Treatment of Colloid Cysts

Colloid cysts are best treated by surgical removal, but sometimes a surgeon will choose to insert a shunt to bypass the cyst. This technique is described in more detail in chapter 11.

Choroid Plexus Papillomas

Choroid plexus papillomas are rare tumors that arise in the choroid plexus, cells in the ventricles of the brain that produce cerebrospinal fluid.

Symptoms of Choroid Plexus Papillomas

Choroid plexus papillomas grow in the ventricles and may cause hydrocephalus either by blocking CSF flow or by secreting too much CSF. The blockage of this fluid creates pressure that can cause headache, dizziness, and nausea.

Diagnosis of Choroid Plexus Papillomas

The initial diagnosis is made by MRI. The scan will show an enhancing mass (that is, a mass that shows up when a contrast agent is given with the MRI) in the ventricle.

Treatment of Choroid Plexus Papillomas

Choroid plexus papillomas are best treated by surgical removal.

Hemangioblastomas

Hemangioblastomas are rare benign tumors composed of cells from the lining of the blood vessels. We most often find them in the cerebellum and the brain stem, but they may also appear in other parts of the brain and spinal cord.

Symptoms of Hemangioblastomas

In the cerebellum, these tumors can block the flow of spinal fluid and can cause unsteadiness. These slowly growing tumors may be a feature of Von Hippel-Lindau disease, an inherited disorder that is associated with retinal angiomas, pancreatic cysts, and kidney cancer (renal cell carcinoma); a patient with a hemangioblastoma should also be screened for these tumors.

Diagnosis of Hemangioblastomas

Either a CT or an MRI scan may confirm the presence of a hemangioblastoma, which usually appears on these scans as an enhancing mass, often with a cyst around it.

Treatment of Hemangioblastomas

Usually we can remove hemangioblastomas through surgery. When they are completely taken out, they do not recur, but if they are incompletely removed, they generally do reappear. Radiosurgery is another treatment for these tumors if they are deep in the brain.

Presently there are clinical trials of anti-angiogenic agents (drugs that cut off the blood supply to these tumors) for patients with hemangioblastomas, but their effectiveness has not been proven.

Dysembryoplastic Neuroepithelial Tumors

Dysembryoplastic neuroepithelial tumors (DNTs) are rare benign tumors, usually in the temporal lobe of children. They are diagnosed by MRI scans and can be treated well with surgery.

Unusual Primary Malignant Brain Tumors

Lymphomas

Primary lymphomas of the central nervous system are tumors of unknown origin that can appear spontaneously or in a patient with some compromise of the immune system—AIDS is one example. They are a little more common in men than in women.

Symptoms of Lymphomas

Lymphomas may produce a "mass effect" (see chapter 2) with headache; sometimes there are psychological changes as well.

Diagnosis of Lymphomas

Lymphomas tend to be enhancing masses on CT and MRI. They resemble gliomas in most respects; an unusual feature is that they may disappear a few days after the patient begins to take steroids.

Treatment of Lymphomas

Lymphomas are usually treated with radiation or chemotherapy. Surgery is generally limited to a biopsy if lymphoma is suspected.

Medulloblastomas

At the age of nine, Charlie had increasingly severe headaches and nausea, and often lost his balance. An MRI at that time showed a mass in his cerebellum—a medulloblastoma. Surgical removal was followed by radiation and chemotherapy. His tumor has never recurred, but he has significant learning disabilities thought to be from his treatment.

Almost one-fifth of all brain tumors that occur in childhood are medulloblastomas. They are more common in boys than in girls, and they tend to occur between the ages of 5 and 9 years. Medulloblastomas are always located in the cerebellum. They usually arise in the middle of the cerebellum in children and in the cerebellar hemisphere in adults. These tumors can grow quickly and spread beyond the brain to other parts of the central nervous system.

Symptoms of a Medulloblastoma

These tumors may cause headaches, vomiting, unsteadiness, and a sense of pressure in the head.

Diagnosis of a Medulloblastoma

We can find medulloblastomas on MRI scans, but as with most brain tumors, a biopsy is necessary to confirm the diagnosis. Under the microscope, medulloblastomas are composed of small round cells that stain blue with our usual stains.

Treatment of a Medulloblastoma

The tendency of medulloblastomas to spread makes it difficult to completely remove them surgically, but the more we can remove, the better. Chemotherapy and craniospinal radiation may be used after surgery to control their metastasis.

We sometimes give chemotherapy to children who are younger than three in order to prolong the period until it is safe to give radiation therapy (see chapter 17).

Primitive Neuroectodermal Tumors

Primitive neuroectodermal tumors are rare, rapidly spreading masses that are most common in children and young adults. They may originate in residual cells from the early growth of the nervous system and are found most often in the cerebral hemispheres. They resemble medulloblastomas in their appearance.

Symptoms of a Primitive Neuroectodermal Tumor

Numbness, weakness, or headaches may occur with these tumors.

Diagnosis of a Primitive Neuroectodermal Tumor

These tumors are diagnosed by MRI scans and biopsy.

Treatment of a Primitive Neuroectodermal Tumor

Complete surgical removal, if possible, followed by radiation and chemotherapy, is the usual course of treatment.

Germ-Cell Tumors

Germ-cell tumors originate in the cells that become eggs or sperm. In the brain, these tumors usually occur near the pineal gland or in the region above the pituitary gland. Types of germ-cell tumors are:

- *Germinoma.* These tumors are the most common germ-cell tumors in the brain.
- *Teratoma.* These rare, benign tumors are usually found in infants. They most often occur in male newborns.
- *Embryonal carcinoma.* This is a very aggressive tumor that tends to metastasize.
- *Choriocarcinoma.* This tumor is made up of cells that normally produce the placenta; it is also very aggressive.
- *Endodermal-sinus (yolk sac) tumors.* Tumors that come from primitive precursor cells and are also very aggressive.

Mixed germ-cell tumors also occur.

Symptoms of Germ-Cell Tumors

These tumors tend to cause headaches and nonspecific symptoms such as uncoordinated muscular movements (*ataxia*).

Diagnosis of Germ-Cell Tumors

Sometimes samples of cerebrospinal fluid (CSF) or blood can lead to a diagnosis of a choriocarcinoma because the level of beta-human chorionic gonadotropin is elevated. Usually, however, biopsy is necessary.

Treatment of Germ-Cell Tumors

Most germ-cell tumors are treated by surgery, radiation, and chemotherapy. Benign tumors such as teratomas should be surgically removed if possible.

Pineal Region Tumors

Terry, a six-year-old boy, was usually very active. About four months ago, he began to complain of headaches and nausea. He would eat and enjoy eating but after that he would throw up. His headaches, which were particularly bad in the morning, grew worse and he began to miss school. An MRI scan showed that part of his problem was excessive fluid in the brain (hydrocephalus) and he had a mass in his pineal gland. A sample of tissue removed during a biopsy confirmed that he had a pineal cell tumor.

The pineal gland sits in the middle of the brain. Pineal tumors are rare in adults, more common in children. They can be divided into two categories—tumors arising from the pineal gland itself and tumors arising in the area of the pineal gland. Pineal tumors include:

- *Pineocytomas:* Grade II pineal tumors that grow slowly
- *Intermediate pineal tumors:* these are halfway between low- and high-grade pineal tumors
- *Pineoblastomas:* aggressive (Grade IV) pineal tumors
- *Astrocytomas* of the pineal region

Germ-cell tumors and meningiomas may grow in this region as well.

Symptoms of Pineal Region Tumors
These tumors present a typical pattern of headache with double vision because they compress the cerebrospinal fluid pathways in the brain.

Diagnosis of Pineal Region Tumors
The diagnosis is made by an MRI scan, which reveals a mass in the pineal gland.

Treatment of Pineal Region Tumors
These tumors are usually treated by surgery followed by radiation and chemotherapy.

Chordomas

Chordomas are slow-growing tumors that most often are detected in people in their twenties and thirties. They are found in the *clivus,* a part of the brain stem; they rarely metastasize.

Symptoms of Chordomas

Advanced chordomas can cause double vision, but usually these tumors do not cause symptoms.

Diagnosis of Chordomas

We can diagnose chordomas by MRI or CT scans.

Treatment of Chordomas

We can treat chordomas with surgery and then radiation. These tumors can recur after treatment.

Choroid-Plexus Carcinomas

Choroid-plexus carcinomas are rare tumors that occur most often in the ventricles in children.

Symptoms of Choroid-Plexus Carcinomas

This type of tumor increases the amount of cerebrospinal fluid (CSF) in the brain (hydrocephalus) so that the intracranial pressure rises. They may also block CSF flow in the brain.

Diagnosis of Choroid-Plexus Carcinomas

Choroid-plexus tumors are diagnosed as masses in the ventricles of the brain by either CT or MRI scans.

Treatment of Choroid-Plexus Carcinomas

We treat choroid-plexus carcinomas with surgery. If the operation is not successful in controlling hydrocephalus, we can also insert a tube called a shunt into the brain to drain cerebrospinal fluid. We follow with radiation in most cases (see chapter 11).

Now that you are familiar with the types of primary tumors (those that arise in the brain itself), let's continue to chapter 6, where we will discuss the symptoms, diagnosis, and treatment of tumors that have spread to the brain from other parts of the body—metastatic brain tumors.

6

■

Metastatic Brain Tumors

Thus far I have talked about the many types of tumors that develop in the brain itself, "primary" brain tumors. In this chapter, I will describe tumors that spread to the brain from cancer in other parts of the body. This chapter is divided into two sections: tumors that occur within the brain and tumors that appear in the lining of the brain, the meninges.

Single and Multiple Metastases to the Brain

> Ralph had lung cancer one year ago and a thoracic surgeon operated to remove the tumor from his lung. At the time, his lymph nodes did not appear to be involved with the cancer. He did well until his leg began to hurt three months ago. A bone scan showed cancer in the long bone of the leg and he had radiation therapy that alleviated his pain. However, his doctor decided to restage his tumor and did an MRI of the head as well as other tests. The MRI revealed that he had a 1-inch mass in his brain. He came to our group to find out about options for treatment.

Symptoms of Metastases

Cerebral metastases are important complications of systemic cancer; they occur in 30 percent of patients with this disease. These tumors can cause headache, gradual weakness, or loss of sensation, or sometimes a stroke with hemorrhage. Tumors that are especially likely to metastasize to the brain are melanoma, breast cancer, small-cell lung cancer, and non-Hodgkin's lymphoma. Brain metastases are becoming a major problem in oncology, generally because the brain is a site where normal chemotherapy does not penetrate. As we develop our ability to control the disease elsewhere in the body, cancer in the brain remains difficult to control. In half of patients with cerebral metastases, metastatic disease is found only in the central nervous system.

Diagnosis of Metastases

We can diagnose metastases in the brain by MRI with contrast enhancement (see chapter 2).

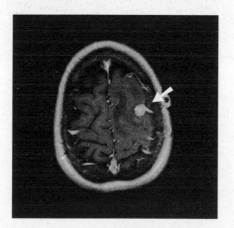 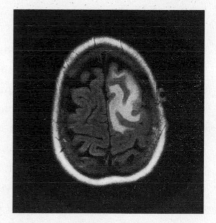

Figures 6-1.A and 6-1.B.   A typical metastasis.

Figure 6-1.A shows the metastasis. Directly over it on the scalp is a "fiducial," a marker placed to help computer registration for localization of the mass for surgery. Figure 6-1.B, done as a FLAIR sequence, shows the swelling (edema) produced by the tumor. In figure 6-1.A, this swelling is seen as a dark area.

Treatment of Metastases

1. *Surgery.* Surgery is the best therapeutic option for single metastatic tumors in most cases. This is especially true if:

- The primary site is unknown.
- The tumor is well controlled in the rest of the body but there is a brain metastasis.
- The metastasis is causing symptoms.

In deciding whether or not to perform surgery, the surgeon will need to weigh the risks of it against its benefits. Generally, however, with image-guided techniques virtually all tumors can be resected (removed surgically).

2. *Radiation.* In the past, whole-brain radiation therapy was usually the primary treatment for brain metastases. It is still used if there are more than three metastases, but this treatment has major side effects in terms of cognitive and other problems. If there is the likelihood of survival beyond one year, these problems can be extremely significant. Survival after whole-brain radiation for metastases is usually 6 to 12 months.

Radiosurgery, a focused form of radiation, is more effective than whole-brain radiation in treating up to three metastatic tumors. It has a 90 percent chance of controlling the metastasis. There is an ongoing discussion about whether whole-brain radiation therapy should be given for metastastic disease; some centers no longer use this therapy because of its long-term consequences, which are discussed in chapter 12.

In general, surgery has a 95 percent chance of controlling metastases (even those tumors in a part of the brain called the eloquent cortex) for the lifetime of the patient. We have shown that with surgery under local anesthesia and guidance techniques we can remove metastases even from the movement, sensory, visual, or speech areas of the brain, with a major likelihood of improvement. One study showed that more than 80 percent of patients got better after surgical resection.

Meningeal Carcinomatosis86

Meningeal carcinomatosis is cancer that is metastatic to the cerebral meninges. As you may recall from chapter 1, the meninges are three sheets of tissue that surround the brain. The first of these sheets is the *pia*, which tightly surrounds the cerebrum and cerebellum. The second is the *arach-*

noid, which is more loosely connected to the skull and contains cerebrospinal fluid (CSF). The third is the *dura,* a very tough outer layer that is tightly connected to the skull.

Meningeal carcinomatosis represents approximately 5 percent of metastatic tumors; breast, lung, and melanoma are the most common primary tumors that produce this problem.

Symptoms of Meningeal Carcinomatosis

Multiple problems with the cranial-nerve and spinal-nerve roots are common presenting syndromes—patients have facial numbness or weakness, double vision, swallowing difficulty, and other problems associated with the cranial nerves.

Diagnosis of Meningeal Carcinomatosis

We can diagnose this condition by looking for malignant cells in the cerebrospinal fluid (CSF) from a sample obtained by a lumbar puncture. Large amounts of CSF must be obtained by lumbar or ventricular puncture to have an adequate sample. We can also make a diagnosis with an MRI using contrast enhancement; this scan may reveal a coating of the meninges of the brain.

Treatment of Meningeal Carcinomatosis

We usually treat this disorder with radiation directed to the brain and spinal cord. We may also deliver chemotherapy to the affected area through a ventricular catheter (see chapter 13).

Brain tumors range from highly curable benign tumors to those that, because of their aggressive nature, may require aggressive treatment. No matter what kind of brain tumor you may be faced with, you probably have questions about whether and how to treat it and how your diagnosis will affect your life and that of your family. If your child has a brain tumor, you will confront another set of challenges. These issues are covered next, in Part Three.

PART THREE

———■———

Living with a
Brain Tumor

Once you have a diagnosis, you must make several important decisions—not just regarding your treatment, although those choices are most important, but about your work, your finances, your family responsibilities, and the way in which a brain tumor will affect your perception of yourself and your relationships. If your child has a brain tumor, you will have another set of issues to consider—again, not just regarding the best course of treatment, but about your child's education, mental health, and his or her growth and development. In Part Three, I will suggest ways to help you find your way through these decisions, and you will meet others who have faced similar challenges.

7

—■—

How to Think about Treatment

"There's an aggressively growing mass in the back of your child's head." It was Mack truck news. We walked numbly to the surgical floor in disbelief.

—Mother of a child with a brain tumor

If you've recently learned that you have a brain tumor, keep this in mind: *You are a statistic of one.* No two tumors are alike. No one else shares your genetic makeup and your unique brain structure. This doesn't mean that you have to face this journey alone. It does mean that as you explore treatment options, treatment centers, and "success rates" of various procedures, you cannot assume that the statistics that you encounter apply to you.

That said, at this point you need to navigate the often confusing rapids of health care options as quickly as you can. Responsive, knowledgeable treatment is key.

You will need to find a doctor who will respect your ideas about treatment, a physician who you can trust. This physician will be your primary source of information and care, but he or she also should work with a group of other highly skilled professionals. Your brain tumor should be managed with a multidisciplinary team. The team that will care for you should work at a hospital or medical center with oncology nurses, pathologists, neurologists, neurosurgeons, radiation oncologists, chemotherapy specialists, and others as needed. This team should be able to answer your questions and offer you the best treatment possible; if they can't, they should be able to refer you to another team that can.

In this chapter, I will include a list of questions you might want to ask your doctor, explain the value of seeking second opinions, and discuss how to work with your health insurance plan. Finally, I will tell you where to look on the Internet to explore the latest research and clinical trials of treatments for the tumor that you must now fight.

What Kind of Treatment Will I Need?

Depending on where your tumor is located, you will most likely need to have an operation to remove it. If you have brain surgery, you will need to take various medications for swelling, seizures, and other complications during the rehabilitative period. You may also require radiation, chemotherapy, and newer therapies such as immunotherapy. You might start with a more conventional form of treatment and then try an experimental therapy, or vice versa. I describe these treatments in detail in Part Four. Table 7-1 outlines factors to consider as you make these important choices.

A good health care team can help you find the best course of treatment, which will depend on:

- Your wishes regarding treatment.
- The type of brain tumor.
- Where the tumor is located.
- The size of the tumor.
- The risks and potential benefits of the available treatment options—no treatment plan is guaranteed.
- Your overall health.
- Your age.
- The type of health care services that are available to you, and your ability to travel to an appropriate center.
- Whether you have family in a part of the country where a particular treatment or clinical trial is being offered.

Each person is like no other, and various treatment methods and clinical trials have different results for different patients, so no doctor can give you a definite answer about what will work for you. Don't pursue treatment with any health care provider who promises a certain cure, but try to find one who views your glass as being half full—and believes that with the best treatment you will do well.

TABLE 7-1

A General Outline of Decisions Regarding Treatment

Imaging shows what appears to be a brain tumor

    a. DECISION 1: Do we watch it, biopsy it, or try to remove it?

After these steps have been carried out

    a. DECISION 2: Do I need further treatment?
       i. Radiation?
      ii. Chemotherapy?
     iii. Should I enter a clinical trial?

If the tumor appears to be coming back

    a. DECISION 3: Usually made later along the tumor course.
       i. Should I enter a clinical trial or use experimental therapy?
      ii. Does surgery or radiation need to be done again?
     iii. Should anything be done at all?

Pros and Cons of Different Kinds of Treatment

One of the first major decisions that patients and physicians face together after the likely diagnosis of a brain tumor is whether to proceed with complete surgical removal of the tumor or whether to have just a biopsy. A biopsy usually involves taking a sample of tumor to find out what it is rather than trying to remove it.

For benign tumors, it is usually best to remove the entire tumor if possible, and even for malignant tumors, surgery to remove the tumor has several advantages over a biopsy. By removing the tumor mass, we can make room to allow for the swelling of the brain tissue that occurs both with radiation therapy and with tumor recurrence. The more tumor we can take out during surgery, the less we will have to treat with other forms of therapy afterward. The larger mass we remove during surgery is also a bigger and better biopsy sample; our ability to diagnose and grade the tumor is improved because we have more cells to examine. Since the cells often vary throughout a brain tumor mass, and a prognosis is based on the part of the tumor with the highest (most malignant) grade, access to more of the tissue provides us with a clearer picture of what the tumor is up to.

The theoretical advantages of surgical removal over biopsy have to be weighed against the added three to four days in the hospital and the possible longer recovery period after surgery. Although no multicenter, randomized, double-blind controlled trials comparing biopsy with surgical removal have been carried out, many oncologists and surgeons believe that it is best to remove a tumor that we can see on imaging studies whenever it is safe to do so.

After the initial surgery, there may seem to be an overwhelming variety of treatment options. I like to think of these as falling into two categories: treatments that are standard and should be pursued, and those that are investigational or experimental. For malignant gliomas, for example, radiation therapy with chemotherapy is the standard treatment at the beginning. It would not be a good idea to neglect this treatment for new and untried treatments at the outset. As the tumor continues to resist some traditional treatments, however, experimental therapies become more reasonable options.

Types of Specialists Who Care for Patients with Brain Tumors

You will encounter many specialists along your journey with a brain tumor. These specialists can give you the most effective, successful care if they're working together as a team.

Neurosurgeons are specialists who operate on the nervous system. They are often the first doctors to see you after the primary care doctor has made a tentative diagnosis, and can act as the initial "quarterback" for care. Neurosurgeons receive six to eight years of additional training after medical school; *neurosurgical oncologists* are neurosurgeons with special training in treating patients with brain tumors.

Oncologists are medical doctors who specialize in the treatment of cancer of all types.

Neuro-oncologists are neurologists or oncologists who treat brain tumors with medication.

Neuropathologists diagnose diseases of the nervous system by looking at the cells obtained in biopsies.

Neuropsychologists have special training in helping individuals with the psychological effects related to a disease of the nervous system.

Neuroradiologists are experts in brain imaging, including CTs, MRIs, and PET or SPECT scans.

Neurologists are trained to diagnose and treat diseases and disorders of the nervous system.

Epileptologists are neurologists who specialize in epilepsy of all kinds, including that caused by brain tumors.

Nurse clinicians have a master's degree in nursing (M.S.N.).

Nurse practitioners have additional training beyond the registered nurse (R.N.) degree and can see patients somewhat independently.

Oncology certified nurses (O.C.N.) have had special training in cancer care.

Finding a Doctor

Your doctor should be your guide through the treatment process, someone you can trust and feel comfortable with. Does he or she listen to you? Answer your questions? Have a way of getting your questions answered?

If you don't know how to find a brain tumor specialist, ask your primary care physician or other doctor you trust; consider another trustworthy source like a nonprofit organization for patients with brain tumors; or ask other patients who have had brain tumors. Patient advocacy groups such as the Brain Tumor Society or the American Brain Tumor Association may be able to help with this. (These organizations are listed in the appendix.)

When you meet a brain tumor specialist for the first time, you may wish to ask him or her (or a nurse who represents the specialist):

- What course of treatment do you recommend? Why?
- What are the risks and benefits of my treatment options?

- How soon should I begin treatment?
- If I need surgery, what do I need to do to prepare for surgery? How long will I be in the hospital? What is the recovery like? What do I need to consider now regarding my long-term recovery process?
- Will I need help with the activities of daily living, physical therapy, or other types of support?
- Which medical centers and physicians have the most expertise in treating this kind of tumor? Who is actively doing research in this area?
- Do you know of any clinical trials that would apply to my case?
- Have any alternative therapies helped patients in my situation? (NOTE: Any time you take herbal treatments, vitamins, or over-the-counter pain relievers like acetaminophen, tell your doctor. Any of these agents can interact with drugs you are taking, and your health care team can advise you in preventing serious side effects.)

The Value of Second Opinions

You are faced with some major decisions and concerns. Ask questions! Keep asking until you get enough answers to guide you along each step of the way, from diagnosis through treatment and recovery.

Some major medical centers offer free or inexpensive second opinions based on a review of the patient's records, pathology reports, and scans. Others will charge a fee to review this information, and this fee is often not covered by insurance.

Second and third opinions can be valuable, but don't spin your wheels and lose time by getting ten opinions. Talk with two doctors and maybe three (as a tie-breaker); then do something. Going from institute to institute can take its toll both in terms of time and energy. Try to make a decision and go with it—and believe that you have made the best choice possible.

Sometimes, even after visiting many treatment centers in search of the "holy grail," you may not find the answer you hoped to hear. For instance, if your mass is too large, you may not find a health care team that will recommend radiation, which could lead to dangerous and debilitating swelling in the brain. Some types of brain surgery may result in loss of speech, understanding, or the ability to walk—or, more important, the loss of your inner dialogue. Finding a physician who will be honest with you about the benefits and risks of treatment is important. If that trusted physician does not give you the answer you wanted to hear, you may want to get one more opinion, and then be willing to modify your point of view if the second physician agrees with the first.

Finding a Hospital

Try to find a medical center that has a finger on the pulse of the latest treatments both nationally and internationally. In the appendix, you will find the Society for Neuro-Oncology's list of brain tumor centers. Your nurse or doctor may be willing to contact specialists in other institutions if you wish to be referred to a larger treatment center. Some centers allow records and films to be sent, although they may wish to repeat some tests. On paper you may appear to be eligible for the treatment they offer, but by the time they see you, your circumstance may have changed to make you ineligible for that particular trial. If you've decided on a particular course of treatment halfway across the country, stay in regular contact with the center before you go to make sure you still qualify for its program. It can help to have one primary contact person at that center.

Some patients ask if it's safe for them to travel by plane to pursue treatment elsewhere. I tell them that the air cabin pressure affects the soft tissues and the nose—not the skull—so in most cases flying is fine. If the expense of flying to another part of the country for treatment seems prohibitive, contact one of the organizations listed under "emergency medical transportation" in the Resources at the end of this book. One of these groups may be able to provide you with free transportation.

Managing Your Care

While you are going through treatment, you may encounter many different health care providers, and you may find it confusing at times to know which one to call. Ask your doctor or nurse (that is, your primary contact):

- Who should I call if I have questions about medication?
- Who should I call if I have a seizure?
- Who should I call about chemotherapy questions?
- About radiation issues?
- About nausea and vomiting?
- About scheduling scans?

You also may find it frustrating to tell your "story" over and over again to each new provider or specialist you meet. Many of my patients find it helpful to keep a notebook that covers all of the basic information about their health. They take the notebook to appointments and offer it to providers who ask for their story from the beginning. This notebook can include:

- Your past medical history (before your brain tumor was discovered), including any history of high blood pressure or other conditions.
- The date of your diagnosis
- The dates of your MRI and CT scans and copies of them
- A list of your doctors
- A list of all medications you have taken (including vitamins, over-the-counter pain relievers, and herbs), with dosages and any side effects experienced
- Your insurance information
- A calendar with your symptoms and upcoming appointments

If you are being cared for in a teaching hospital, you may meet several residents who want to know about your case. Trainees often provide an important backup for the attending physicians. Nevertheless, going over your story again and again can be draining, so you should ask if they will review your notebook and the chart first and then ask questions.

What about Health Insurance?

If You Have Health Insurance

Contact the member services group at your insurer to find out what kind of coverage you have. A *point of service* (POS) plan is a managed care plan that will allow you to go to physicians and hospitals outside the "network" for a higher charge. A *preferred provider organization* (PPO) is a managed care plan in which care is mostly restricted to a network of health providers and hospitals. It will cost significantly more to use services outside of this network.

In addition to knowing which type of plan you have, call your insurance company to ask:

- Are experimental drugs and procedures covered? Some of the latest techniques in treating brain tumors (such as functional MRI), which are still considered experimental by many insurance agencies, are not covered.
- Are integrative (also called complementary) therapies such as massage, acupuncture, and reiki (a therapy that draws on energy in and around the body; see chapter 18) covered?
- Is physical therapy covered? Some insurers will only cover physical therapy for two weeks.
- What kinds of disability benefits are offered? Some patients find that these benefits are hard to come by, especially if they experience occasional seizures and weakness, but on the outside, they look just fine.

Talk with your health care team and your hospital business office about how you might be able to augment your insurance coverage if necessary. Your hospital social worker is also knowledgeable about these issues, programs, and entitlements, and can help you access what you need and determine your eligibility.

Your physician's office can be helpful in writing letters of appeal to your insurance company if need be. If you find yourself in conflict with your insurance company, or for further guidance from attorneys and case managers in sorting out your benefits, go to www.healthinsuranceinformation.net or contact the nonprofit organization Patient Advocate Foundation (www.patientadvocate.org or 866-512-3861). This foundation may be able to help you apply for Social Security disability, Medicare, Medicaid, and other programs.

If you have health insurance through your job, you may be concerned about what will happen to that coverage if you have to take a leave of absence or if you will no longer be able to work. If you are enrolled in a health plan through your work (in a company of 20 people or more), you may be eligible for COBRA (coverage mandated by the Consolidated Omnibus Budget Reconciliation Act). If you lose your job or change jobs, you may receive short-term (18–36 months) health coverage benefits through this program. To find out more about COBRA, go to www.dol .gov/ebsa/faqs/faq_consumer_cobra.html.

Another useful vehicle for protecting your health benefits falls under the Health Insurance Portability and Accountability Act (HIPAA). This legal protection, which is also called the Kennedy-Kassebaum Act, can help you retain your health coverage through your employer or through a private health insurance plan. For more information, go to www.dol.gov/ ebsa/faqs/faq_consumer_hipaa.html.

If You Do Not Have Health Insurance

You may be able to pay for your care through a government- or pharmaceutical-sponsored program. Resources such as Needy Meds, which provides information about various types of patient-assistance programs, are listed in the Resources section at the end of this book.

Government-funded health insurance plans include:

- *Medicaid,* which covers some medical expenses for people with low income and disabilities. The benefits vary by state. To find out if you qualify for Medicaid, contact your local Department of Welfare or Social Services, or go to www.cms.gov/medicaid.
- *Medicare,* which provides health insurance for people aged 65 and older and some younger patients with disabilities, including blindness and kidney failure. Medicare Part A covers hospital, skilled nursing, home health, and hospice care. Medicare Part B covers outpatients' doctor and hospital visits and some medical equipment and supplies. For more information about Medicare, go to www.cms.gov/medicare.
- *The Hill-Burton Free Medical Care Program,* which provides free or low-cost medical care for people with limited incomes. Not all hospitals participate in this federal program. To find out more, call 800-638-0742 or go to http:www.hrsa.gov/osp/dfcr/about/aboutdiv.htm.

In addition to coverage for your health care costs, you should also explore the resources that will be available to you in the event you have a long recovery period ahead. Ask someone in the human resources department where you work about your company's disability benefits (both short- and long-term).

If you own your home, check with your mortgage company to ensure that you have insurance to cover your house payments if you are unemployed for a while.

You may also be eligible for disability benefits through Social Security. Contact the Social Security Administration at 800-772-1213 or www .socialsecurity.gov. Find out if you qualify for either Social Security disability insurance (SSDI) or supplemental security income (SSI). SSDI is generally available for individuals who have paid Social Security taxes while employed and who expect to be out of work because of a health problem for a year or more. SSI is available to individuals with limited incomes who face blindness or disability, regardless of their employment history. If you qualify for SSI, you may also be eligible for Medicaid coverage of your health care costs.

Where to Find Legitimate Information on the Internet

The Internet can be scary. Before I do a search I always stop to remind myself that everyone's situation is different.
—Woman with an astrocytoma

Many resources are available on line, but it's crucial to visit only responsible Web sites that offer you a balanced picture, not sites that offer you an expensive miracle cure. Be wary of any information that is more than a few years old, even if it's from a respected source. Things are changing in medicine all the time, and yesterday's information may no longer apply. Older studies and advice may not reflect what's happening in brain tumor science today.

When you surf the Web looking for information about managing a brain tumor, you might want to use the following list to help you weigh the legitimacy of a given site:

1. Can you access the site without providing your personal information or a credit card number?
2. Does the site clearly state the source of the medical information it

provides? Does it cite legitimate medical journal articles or give the name and institution of the physician who provides the information?

3. Does the site contain a privacy statement?
4. Does the site contain hostile or offensive language?
5. Does the site endorse a particular drug, therapy, physician, or institution? If so, is the pharmaceutical or institutional support of the site clearly stated?
6. Does the site promote one form of therapy over another, or does it present a broad overview of available treatments?

If you are trying to make a decision about treatment, I would encourage you to bring the information you find on the Internet to your doctor. He or she can help you determine which options are credible and worth pursuing. Your health care team may also provide you with Web site links or telephone numbers for other health centers that are running clinical trials or offering therapies with which they are familiar.

The following is a short list of Web sites I recommend. Other sites that may be helpful are listed at the end of this book.

- **The National Cancer Institute (NCI):** Offers the most comprehensive guide to treatments for brain tumors, www.cancernet.nci.nih.gov. You can also check individual hospital sites for information about their clinical trials and request that they e-mail you when new trials come up. National Cancer Institute Clinical Trial Page: www.cancer.gov/clinical_trials/.
- **Medline:** This database, produced by the National Library of Medicine, is useful for searching through published articles in the medical literature, www.nlm.nih.gov/medlineplus/. **PubMed** is the system that helps you access this information: www.pubmed.org.
- **Brain Tumor Foundation:** www.braintumorfoundation.org.
- **American Brain Tumor Association**: www.abta.org.
- **CANHELP:** A nonprofit organization that offers information about alternative therapies, www.canhelp.com.
- **Brain Tumor Society:** www.tbts.org.
- **Musella Foundation:** musella@virtualtrials.com.
- **National Brain Tumor Foundation:** www.braintumor.org.

Clinical Trials

Many of the major hospitals for adults in the United States that offer sophisticated treatment for brain tumors belong to one of two clinical trial consortiums—the North American Brain Tumor Coalition (NABTC) and the New Approaches to Brain Tumor Therapy (NABTT) Consortium. Children's hospitals may belong to the Children's Oncology Group. Enrollment in clinical trials may be limited. Some hospitals will pay for you and your family to travel to their center for care. They may also cover the cost of your hotel and food. To learn more about clinical trials, see chapter 14.

As you think about treatment for your brain tumor, remember that Lewis and Clark didn't know what they were going to find when they set out on their journey. Still, they relied on their available resources and were open to new ways of doing things along the way. Find a capable physician to guide you and then trust that you will find the answers and outcomes that you are looking for.

In the next chapter, I will tell you about ways in which my patients have prepared themselves for the road ahead.

8

■

What a Brain Tumor Means
for Me and My Family

The shock has been enormous. I have spent many hours wandering around starting to make cups of tea or fill the dishwasher and then just forgetting that I had started. And the fear, for some days, was paralyzing. I often had the urge just to lie down and sleep. But, as the days have gone by, I have my nerve again. Talking and talking, to friends, family, and anyone who would listen has helped. All the statistics in the world will not tell them what is going to happen to me, and I am grateful for the uncertainty and hope that provides.

—Ivan Noble, BBC reporter

Life changes on a dime.

—Amy Masso, a patient with a mixed oligoastrocytoma

Blindsided.

—Meningioma patient, asked to describe her
reaction to her diagnosis in one word

The discovery of a brain tumor is a life-changing event that happens quickly, and for most people there is a surreal quality to the experience, even after a decision has been made about the best course of treatment. The wife of one of my patients couldn't believe that her husband's tumor was real until he began to lose his hair with radiation therapy. The rest of his life was as normal as it had always been: he was still working, going out with friends, and coaching their son's soccer team.

Although the discovery of a brain tumor can be a transformative event regardless of the outcome, some tumors may require no treatment at all. You and your family will have to live with the tumor as you have regular MRI scans to keep an eye on it. In chapter 10, I'll tell you more about strategies for coping in this "watching and waiting" situation.

If your brain tumor requires surgical removal, getting through the operation is often straightforward—many of the difficult issues appear afterward. What other treatments are necessary? Is it ever going to come back? Am I going to be any different in my day-to-day work? If the tumor has metastasized from cancer elsewhere in your body or if it is a primary tumor that turns out to be malignant, you will confront another set of fears and issues around treatment.

No matter what kind of brain tumor you have, its discovery and its effect on your life can have a dramatic impact on the lives of your spouse, children, and extended family. I've seen families torn apart by the long-term disability produced by a tumor and I've seen others rise to a new level in the same circumstance. This chapter will explore some of the issues and concerns that you may face and provide resources to help you and your family address them.

Breaking the News: Telling Others about Your Diagnosis

Discussing your diagnosis with others can become an additional emotional ordeal. In most cases, people won't know what to say at first, so you may have to help them out. That said, as with every other aspect of this journey, don't feel you have to go through this alone. If you find yourself at a loss for words, ask a close friend, nurse, or hospital social worker to help you talk with others about what you are going through

Your Family

> *John was like an intermediary for me. He helped me to hear some things that were harsh. Sometimes I wanted John to talk to the doctors about the harsh realities. Then he would talk to me later at home about it.*
>
> —Christine Hammock, discussing her husband's role in
> *An Open Approach to Living with Cancer*

You can choose how much information you want your family to know about your diagnosis. If you find it difficult to talk with them directly, ask your doctor, nurse, or social worker to meet with all of you.

Some people don't like to think in terms of textbook statistics; others cling to them as a way of framing their experience. I think it's important to remember that there is always hope; some people always do better than the numbers. If you would rather not ask your health care team about your prognosis, but your family wants to know more, ask your doctor or nurse to discuss that information with them when you are out of the room.

Your Children

Your first instinct may be to protect your children from the news of your diagnosis. I try to discourage that, because most children know more about what's going on than we think. They are savvy to life's realities through phone conversations they have overheard and even television shows they have watched. Without true information from the people they trust the most, early on, they can be terrified by what they suspect might be true, especially if a parent's symptoms are progressing and they have no context for knowing what to expect.

Be honest with your children. Keep the door open to conversation so that they will ask questions. Create a climate in your family where the child is not afraid to ask questions, because very often the child's fantasies will be far worse than reality. If (s)he finds that asking questions makes grown-ups uneasy, (s)he may stop asking and persist in being terrified. Of course, you should give due consideration to the age and developmental capacities of the child. A teenager or adolescent can understand a lot more than a three-year-old who may only be able to grasp that a parent is sick.

As a general rule, if children can formulate the question, they can handle—and indeed need—the answers in order to make sense of what is happening. The answers should be simple and to the point—there's no need to give a drawn-out, complicated explanation that may overwhelm your child. When (s)he is ready to process more, (s)he will ask more questions.

Children need to trust their parents to tell the truth, even about the unknowns that your family is facing. Reassure them that everyone is doing what they can to fight the brain tumor. Younger children may have fantasies that this could also happen to the other parent, or to themselves, or that they are in some way responsible. If these concerns do arise, the parent needs to reassure the child otherwise.

Children should get information with respect to their age and based on what is known. Early on, before you have received the results from your biopsy, you may not need to scare your children with the words *brain tumor*. Nevertheless, your children will know that something is wrong. You might say, "Mom is sick and the doctors are running all kinds of tests to find out why. They'll have to do an operation to find out what the problem is and as soon as we find out what it is we will tell you."

If you are concerned about telling your children by yourself, ask a mental health professional who is experienced in working with children to talk with your family. You might also ask your social worker, nurse, or doctor to provide information about your illness and answer any questions your children have. It may be easier, at some point during these meetings, if you leave the room so that your children can ask questions without fear of hurting you. A counselor can talk with them about what to expect and can empower them by teaching them how to respond (for instance, they can explain what a seizure is, what it looks like, and how to call 911 if a parent has one).

Once the initial news has been broken, your health care team at the hospital may be able to recommend a counselor who lives closer to your family so that help is accessible. They may also be able to recommend a music or art therapy program that can help your children express what they may not be able to articulate in words.

Some programs, such as TOPS (Teens of Parent Survivors), are geared specifically for older children. For more information, contact: www.brain trust.org.

Your Friends

Communicating each development to your friends can take on a life of its own and can consume a considerable amount of time and energy, regardless of whether the news is good or bad. Some of my patients establish e-mail, telephone, or letter chains to their friends, family members, colleagues, and church to quickly communicate the essential facts of what's going on. That way, they are spared the burden of calling everyone (or calling everyone back) to repeat the same story over and over again.

A family member who is managing this "communication tree" for you can inform people if you've had an operation, when you will be home, and what your family does or doesn't need (like food or flowers). You may also wish to create a private Web page through www.carepages.com. This free service allows you to provide frequent progress reports to enrolled family and friends and receive tremendous support in the form of posted messages.

It's perfectly okay to ask friends not to call or stop by if you're not feeling up to it. One of my patients advises others: "Know when to say when. If you're tired, feel free to say no. Know your body and its limits." Let your friends know the best time of day to call, if you want them to call you. If you're not up to phone calls, and not up to going online yourself, you can ask a family member to read e-mail messages to you when you are ready to hear them.

E-mail is also a good way to let people know that you care about what's going on with them—you don't want your tumor to be the focus of every conversation and exchange that you have.

How a Brain Tumor May Affect Your Everyday Life

Your Work

If you can keep working, you may find that you're not as adept at dealing with numbers as you used to be, or you may find you can't do as many tasks at once. It can help to write everything down. Consider talking with a professional and having some behavioral neuropsychiatric testing done to identify where your difficulties are and to find strategies for coping with them.

The worst-case scenario, in terms of work, is to be dismissed and lose your health benefits because you can't do the job. If you find that you're really struggling, it may be better to go on disability so that you can keep your health insurance.

As I mentioned in the last chapter, from the outset you should find out what kind of coverage you have through your insurance company. For expenses that are not covered, or if you will need additional financial assistance, talk with the business office of your hospital or contact a nonprofit organization such as the American Cancer Society (800-227-2345) about other sources of coverage.

If your spouse isn't working already, he or she may want to seek a part-time job that offers health benefits and generous leave.

If you need to take a break from work for a while, you may suffer not just from the loss of income, but from the daily outlet for your creativity, intelligence, and usefulness. The loss of a job also can shake your sense of identity if you are the breadwinner. Often this can lead to depression and tension in a family.

Consider ways to keep your creative energy flowing. For instance, after surgery to remove an anaplastic oligodendroglioma, Scott Leaver took a month off from his job as a computer consultant. While he waited to find out what kind of further treatment he would need, he began to paint abstract portraits of his Swiss mountain dog, Lucy. His paintings soon gained admirers and commissions, and his artwork became a second career.

Many patients have told me that their brain tumor, whether benign or malignant, refocused their lives and allowed them to work on what they thought was important. Some people choose to stay at work because it gives their life structure; others prefer to stop working. There isn't a right or wrong answer. Your own circumstances and needs will shape this decision.

Driving

> I missed driving more than expected. I would have liked not to have to rely on others all the time. It gave my friends a way to help—but I would have liked to help my family by being able to drive. Looking back, losing the ability to drive most directly affected my independence.
> —Christine Hammock, *An Open Approach to Living with Cancer*

If you are at risk for seizures, you may have to stop driving for your own safety and that of others. This can be especially challenging for people who have children or grandchildren who depend on them for transportation. If you need to stop driving for a while, try to go along if someone else is doing the driving chores. You will thus feel less isolated and frustrated by this restriction.

Your Home Life

You may wish to make some changes to your house or apartment to help you remain as independent as possible. For instance, some people find it easier to convert a room on the first floor of their house into a bedroom than to depend on others to help them go upstairs while they are regaining their strength after surgery. Other people need a wheelchair ramp into their homes.

Ask your health care team if they can give you a "prescription" to have a rehab consultant visit your home to make an evaluation and recommend possible structural changes. Some insurance companies will cover part of the expense of hiring contractors or installing a stair-lift system.

How Your Tumor May Affect Your Relationships

Your Marriage

> *I've learned to keep my foot on the gas—which is love.*
> —Amy Masso

A brain tumor can present a turning point in a marriage. For some, particularly for those whose relationships were fragile before the diagnosis, the stress can create a wedge that may be difficult to overcome. Others find that this crisis pulls them together—they may choose to marry or to renew marriage vows. Amy Masso, a vibrant young mother, found that her love for and from her husband and child gave her the power to keep going in her fight with a brain tumor.

Ideally, a brain tumor will bring couples together, but it can just as easily—and understandably—push them apart. Your partner may struggle with his or her own emotions. There is grief over the normal life that has been lost and anger that you may no longer be able to drive, work, or help out at home. At times the assumption of extra responsibilities can seem like too much for one person. Your partner may feel resentful because of these added burdens—and then feel guilty for feeling resentful. The milieu of emotions may prove overwhelming for some.

A brain tumor can also place strains on a relationship if you are directing anger and frustration, perhaps unwittingly, toward those around you.

The effects of a tumor on the brain may alter behavior. You may be less inhibited, your sense of humor may change, you may be less empathetic or angrier or more lethargic than usual. Your partner may feel you are so different now that you are not the person he or she married. If your partnership was rocky before the diagnosis, the stress of the illness may make things worse. Even if you have weathered many crises together before, you've probably never experienced anything quite like this. Counseling may help you and your partner deal with fear, resentment, and other difficult emotions.

Partners often express profound sadness at seeing a loved one suffer. One husband said, "I wish I hated her so I didn't have to see her go through this."

It is also important for the person who is healthy to have permission to think about himself, to get out, and do whatever helps him feel whole again.

Your Children

Many children, when faced with a parent's illness, will regress a whole stage. Very young children who have just been potty trained may go back to needing diapers. Children of elementary school age may suspect that something is wrong, but they may not want to ask or they may not know how to ask. They may act out by pushing someone on the playground— it's a cause-and-effect action that they have some control over. Teenagers may begin to act like preadolescents, reacting by talking back at home or acting out in school.

These reactions are all normal, and such behavioral outbursts can be difficult to live with. Donna Dello Iacono, a nurse in our brain tumor group, points out that children should be given some leeway in terms of their behavior in these stressful times. Sometimes it is best to let someone else assume the role of disciplinarian while you are going through treatment.

You can help your children by making it safe to talk about what is happening to you and your family. They need to know that nothing they are doing or feeling is causing your illness—or will make it go away.

Again, look for a counselor who will address your symptoms head on and teach your children how to respond to the changes in your life in a way that keeps you as connected as possible. If you need to sleep a lot, for instance, your children may need to know that it's okay to curl up and take a nap with you. If your family finds strength in religious convictions, you may wish to enlist a priest, rabbi, or other religious counselor who can add a spiritual perspective to your family's experience. Always assure your children that it's okay to ask questions.

If you need to go into the hospital for an extended time, this may be the perfect time for a favorite aunt to come for a visit.

If you work with children as a teacher, you might ask your hospital social worker to come to school to explain your illness to the children in your class.

Although none of us can prepare completely for what life has in store, we can all cope better when we have some idea of what to expect.

How a Brain Tumor May Affect Your Sense of Self

Your Self-Identity

The physical experience of a brain tumor can certainly be difficult, and if you have this illness you may also be in for a wrenching emotional time. As with any crisis, you may go through a process of grieving for the life you have lost, acceptance, and adjustment. Many people work through their shock and anger without significant psychological effects, yet others suffer more intense emotional damage that can result in long-lasting personal or marital problems.

In her "crisis theory," professor and social worker Lydia Rapoport suggests that a crisis can be seen as a threat, a loss, or a challenge. The diagnosis of a brain tumor is certainly a crisis; if it is perceived as a threat it can be met with anxiety; as a loss it can be met with depression; but if it is perceived as a challenge, a person can mobilize his or her energy and problem-solving skills. Paul Faircloth, a social worker at our hospital, notes, "You do see different responses. Some folks might search the Web and all of their contacts, and go from center to center to see which clinical trials might be available—looking for the best possible treatment. Others withdraw in the face of this diagnosis into a depression. A lot depends on their underlying personality, their inner strengths and resources, and social support from their family and friends."

A brain tumor can radically change your self-identity. Even if your tumor is removed and you are doing well, you may continue to see yourself as someone who is very different from other people. In chapter 18, I'll tell you how some of my patients have come to terms with both their physical and emotional scars.

Even as your identity is challenged, you'll find remarkable capacities to maintain your strength, your resolve, and your underlying sense of self. A person with a brain tumor can face tremendous losses: health, functioning, independence, job, financial security, roles within the family, relationships, favorite pastimes, sports, driving, intellect, and expectations for a long healthy life. These devastating losses can affect the very core of your being. "Yet even as a person's roles and responsibilities may change," Faircloth suggests, "it's also important to look at what remains: the ability to laugh, to feel, to think, to enjoy a grandchild, and the freedom to choose how to deal with the situation. Two things that amaze me about brain tumor patients are the strengths and abilities they have that they didn't realize they had. They have to draw on their inner resources. One's mind doesn't want to go there. But when forced to go there because it is happening to them, they find inner strengths and external strengths [from their support system of family and friends]. It's truly amazing how resilient people are. They find the strength within themselves and their loved ones to endure."

As you wrestle with your shock, anger, and disbelief—and your fear of the unknown—many resources are available to help, including family members, physicians, counselors, mental health professionals, social workers, clergy, local and national support groups, hospital-sponsored support groups, Internet information pages and talk groups, and hotlines. Talk with your health care team about the resources they recommend, and look through the Resources section at the end of this book.

Coping

As brain tumor survivors we are all warriors, heroes, fighting our battles each day. Every day brings challenges, and meeting them is your goal. Nowhere does it say that this is going to be easy or that you have to be happy and smiling all the time. You are not expected to.

As you go through surgeries and other treatments, you and

your family will meet up with the "new" you. Accepting this "new" you and leaving behind the old you will be difficult. You will get through that, be patient. It is a difficult challenge, but you will all get there.

There really has been no secret to my success in my long-term survivorship. I sure have kicked the statistics, though. I have always been in attack mode. The need to be in control of my tumor, to be assertive, to be proactive instead of reactive has always been my way. Education has always empowered me, top on my list. Attending conferences and asking questions are very important, and attending support groups regularly, even during treatment, helped me get through my most difficult, trying times.

—Sheryl Shetsky, president, Florida Brain Tumor Association

Having a brain tumor is like finding yourself in the middle of a dark forest. You're not sure how you got there, and you don't know how you'll get out. Reach out to your family, your friends, and other supportive people. They can help you find your way out of the darkness one step at a time.

A Little Help from Your Friends (and Family)

Friends may want to help by feeding you and your family. Let them. They may want to provide transportation for you or your family. Let them. They may want to include you in their prayer list. Let them. You may want to ask a friend or family member to coordinate those efforts so that you aren't inundated with food one day and not covered at all another. He or she can take care of communicating your family's preferences and any allergies or other restrictions you may have.

When you ask for help, be specific. If a friend asks if there is anything that he can do for you, he means it! He will probably be relieved if you make a specific request (for instance, to take a package to the post office). Some people aren't sure what to do if a person says that he or she doesn't need anything.

Don't be surprised if your relationships change at this time. The people you've always relied on, the ones you always believed would be there no matter what, may suddenly seem unavailable. The situation is overwhelming for them. Others whom you barely know may step forward and be very present for you. Perhaps they have been through a similar experience or care about someone else who has.

It may help to have a "paid friend," a social worker or other counselor who can listen objectively. It may be easier for you to talk with such a person without feeling guilty that you are imposing your suffering on those you love.

Counselors

> *Feel it, acknowledge it, and let it go.*
>
> —Amy Masso

A brain tumor is unlike any other health problem. If you lose a breast or even a leg, you can still function and the person you are inside remains intact. Yet because the brain controls your physical, psychological, and emotional nature, a brain tumor and its treaments can truly change who you are. You may lose your early memories or only have memories of the past. Depending on the area of the brain where the tumor is, you also may experience euphoria, absence of feeling (flat affect), impatience, anger, and depression. These personality changes can be quite difficult for you and your family to adjust to.

A person with short-term memory loss may swing from complaining of a "number 10" headache (on a scale of 1 to 10, 10 being the most extreme) to a euphoric sense that all is well. The antithesis of this problem, and one of the hardest states of mind to deal with, is no mood at all. You may completely lack motivation to get up, get dressed, eat, or take care of yourself. Small tasks like taking out the trash may feel overwhelming.

Even though you and your family are clearly in the throes of a crisis because of your tumor, you may find yourself yelling at the dog and the children and wonder why you are doing it. You may find yourself slipping into depression and trying to cope by drinking or self-medicating with other substances. Ask your health care team if it is normal for you to be feeling like this. You may wish to see a counselor to talk about the stresses you are facing. Depending on the severity of your mood swings, a psychiatrist can work with your physician to prescribe a mood-stabilizing drug or antidepressant that can help.

Many of my patients feel they can manage on their own because they have dealt with other crises in their lives, and resist seeing a counselor at first. I usually advise my patients to try a visit with this type of professional once. Usually, if they go once, they keep going back. It's such a relief to be able to set down your burdens, even for an hour. You don't want depression to be the focus of your life, just as you don't want your tumor to be. But if you can talk about it, you can cope with it and the rest of your life will be better.

Mental Health Professionals

The terms *psychiatrist, psychologist,* and *social worker* may be loaded with stigma for you, but these professionals have worked with many other people who share your situation and they really can help. Your doctor or nurse can recommend such a counselor at the center where you are receiving treatment. If you live far away from the hospital, your primary care physician can refer you to a mental health professional in your community. The beauty of meeting with a counselor is that you don't have to protect what you say. During psychotherapy, or "talk" therapy, you can vent your anger, frustration, and grief over the loss of your normal life— without concerns about upsetting your family and friends.

You may also wish to pursue group psychotherapy with a mental health counselor or a support group, through either a local or national nonprofit organization such as the Brain Tumor Society or a hospital-based group. Social worker Paul Faircloth says that in the brain tumor support groups that he has co-led with Nancy Olsen Bailey, R.N., people tend to say things that they couldn't say with others who would not or might not understand. He also notes that often members of these groups share a sense of humor that they can hardly express elsewhere. "It can be quite striking in the group and the depth of understanding and support can be quite unique." See chapter 18 and the Resources section for more information about these groups.

Clergy

Many centers that treat people with brain tumors have priests, rabbis, and other clergy on staff to counsel patients and their families. Some patients find comfort in religion and focus on the relationship between faith and healing. For many patients, the brain tumor makes them truly understand "one day at a time"—gratitude for each day and the hope that it will bring health and healing. They also learn the importance of healthy selfishness—asking for guidance or healing, and trying to be sure your needs are met as well as the needs of those around you.

Taking Care of Yourself

While you are wrestling with decisions about treatment and making plans for how to care for your family during your recuperation, don't forget to eat, sleep, and take care of yourself in general. Outlets such as music, art, and dance—anything you enjoy that can make you feel most like yourself—can help at this time. People deal with things differently. As Sheryl Shetsky says to other people who are fighting brain tumors, "Don't try to get back to who you were then. This is likely a new and improved you in many ways; moving on is the way to go."

9

■

Raising a Child Who Has a Brain Tumor

When he was two, he woke up one day with a head tilt. The pediatrician thought he might have wax in his ears. When he didn't improve, we took him to an orthopedist, who put him in a neck brace. Then we went to an optometrist—we thought maybe one eye was weaker than the other. In fact, he had a lump the size of a golf ball in his cerebellum.

In fairness, the location of the tumor made it difficult to diagnose without a scan. He did not have the classic symptoms of a brain tumor at first—no vomiting or headache. He was eating and sleeping normally. Then, as the mass grew and the amount of fluid in his brain increased, he began to vomit. He was walking like a drunken sailor by the time a pediatric neurologist ordered a CT scan.

—Mother of a child with a brain tumor

The Central Brain Tumor Registry of the United States estimates that 3,410 new cases of primary brain and central nervous system tumors were diagnosed in children in the United States in 2005. This number includes both benign and malignant tumors. Of these, approximately 2,590 occurred in children who were younger than age fifteen. Fortunately, new surgical techniques and developments in chemotherapy and radiation treatments in recent years have improved the prognosis for many of them. In chapter 17, I will describe these and other treatment options for children.

In this chapter, you will find information about other issues involved with raising a child who has a brain tumor. For instance, you may wonder how to talk with your child about the diagnosis and the treatment ahead of him. Brothers and sisters will be affected by this crisis in the family.

After your child's surgery or other treatment, you may face other issues regarding reentry into school. Just like adults, elementary school-age children, teenagers, and young adults will all have to come to terms with their new identity and the challenges of living with a brain tumor.

Talking with Your Child

If possible, talk with your child's doctor about the best way to explain the diagnosis and treatment of your child's brain tumor. Children usually sense when something is wrong, and should not be left to provide their own answers using often overactive imaginations. Explaining the diagnosis becomes more urgent if the child requires an operation, in which case he or she needs to be told ahead of time about hospitalization.

Tish Reidy, a nurse practitioner in neurosurgery at Children's Hospital in Boston, suggests that it may be best to avoid terms like "cancer," "malignant," and "benign" when describing a brain tumor diagnosis to a child. Depending on the child's age, it is okay to explain that he has a "lump" in his head and that the doctors will do something to fix his headaches or other relevant symptoms. Use simple language to explain what scanners (and sometimes radiotherapy) devices do; for example, children who undergo radiation therapy can be told that a powerful x-ray is going to zap the bad cells.

Christopher Turner, M.D., director of outcomes research for pediatric neuro-oncology at the Dana-Farber/Children's Hospital Cancer Center in Boston, encourages parents to tailor their discussions to the developmental level of the child. A five-year-old and a thirteen-year-old will have different needs. "Many parents do not feel comfortable talking to their children about a potentially life-threatening disease such as having a brain tumor," Turner says. "We have trained pediatric psychologists and social workers who are part of the team to help families address these issues."

One such psychologist is Gerald Koocher, Ph.D., dean and professor at the School for Health Studies at Simmons College in Boston. He has worked with many families in this situation, and he urges parents to keep the door to conversation open so that the child feels comfortable talking about his fears. For example, you might say to your child, "When you are feeling angry or unhappy you can tell us because we feel the same way and we're not afraid to talk about those feelings." Koocher recommends that parents talk with a mental health professional who is trained in working with children. A child should be given "clarity of communication in a way that lets him express his fears and concerns." This openness assures the child that he will have his medical needs taken care of and the people he cares about will not abandon him.

Wondering Why

Parents tend to ask their own, very natural questions early on: Why did this happen to my child? Was it something I did? Was it because I didn't eat the right food or because I exercised when I was pregnant? I live in a town where four other kids have brain tumors. Is it something in the environment?

"Unfortunately," Dr. Turner notes, "for the vast majority of brain tumors, there is no answer to those questions."

The Rest of the Family

When my whole family came to visit me for my birthday, I sat in a wheelchair and gazed at them, feeling splendid. I could tell they were shocked at the sight of me. I had been an absolutely normal nine-year-old the last time they saw me, some ten days before. My older sister spoke politely to me, as did my twin sister. They'd never been polite to me before, and I knew that a chasm had opened between us. How could I explain that the way I felt now was actually better? How could they ever know where I had just come from? Suddenly I understood the term visiting. I was in one place, they were in another, and they were only pausing. We made polite conversation about people at school, from the neighborhood, talked about things entirely inconsequential because it wasn't the subject that counted but the gesture of conversation itself. You could have parsed each sentence not into nouns and verbs but into signs and symbols, artificial reports from a buffer zone none of us really owned or cared to inhabit.

—Lucy Grealy, *Autobiography of a Face*

Having one child with a brain tumor is obviously traumatic for both the child and his or her parents. All families had lives before the brain tumor was discovered, and parents may have difficulty taking time off from work to go back and forth to the hospital. Some struggle to remain employed. Siblings are also affected, both by the concern for their brother or sister and the absence of their parents (who may be staying overnight at the hospital). Sometimes a social worker, psychologist, or psychiatrist can help families who are facing these issues.

If your child has surgery, brothers and sisters generally should not visit in the intensive care unit, but they may be able to visit when he or she is on a regular hospital floor. Many pediatric floors have playrooms that can be therapeutic both for the child who is ill and his or her siblings.

Going Home

After treatment, most younger children do better at home. They are usually highly motivated to get out of the hospital and get back to the normal business of childhood—play.

If your child has been out of school for some time, ask your health care team if someone from the hospital can come to her school for a visit. At the Dana-Farber Cancer Institute, the back-to-school team includes the child's pediatric psychologist, school specialists, and a "child life" person (also called a play therapist). This team first meets and talks with the student/patient and her parent. Then they visit the child's school either before the child returns or during her first day back to school. They explain where the child has been and answer questions from the other kids in the class.

Children who are in the middle of their therapy have a special set of issues to work through when they go back to school. If they have additional chemotherapy and radiation, for instance, they may lose their hair, lose weight, and may look different. Again, a team from the hospital can work with the teacher and the child's classmates to address these changes.

Going back to school is usually pleasurable for the child. Often the class has been supportive through his or her absence, and classmates are missed so much that the child is eager to return to school to see them. Going back brings more normalcy to the child's life than sitting at home. "Most kids want to be in school," Turner says. "It's the child's social environment that he or she feels comfortable with. Most kids want to get back to their normal routine and surroundings."

Growing Up with a Brain Tumor

He didn't talk about his experience with peers until he was in third grade. By the time he was nine, he began to realize that other people had different types of cancer, and he was lucky to survive. He wondered how his cancer was different from others.
— Mother of a child with a brain tumor

Some pediatric brain tumor centers have a school liaison program. When the child has completed treatment in the hospital, these programs give the child a formal neurocognitive evaluation that focuses on areas in which she is strong and not so strong. The school liaison team then takes the report from this evaluation and works with the child's school to create an educational plan (either a "504" or an individual education plan, an IEP).

This neuropsychological assessment is particularly important for children who do not have any obvious impairments such as blindness or deafness. Sometimes treatment for a brain tumor can result in a subtle language-processing problem that might be mistaken by a teacher for laziness or inattention.

School systems vary widely. Some will bend over backward to support children and give them the services they need; other systems, because of a scarcity of resources, fail to provide them. Others are well meaning but need some guidance from professionals, as they might never have worked with a child in a similar situation previously. Many times families must be their child's advocate in seeking services from schools. In rare cases, such advocacy is to no avail. In such instances, parents may have to resort to the legal system (that is, sue the school system) or move to another town just to get the support services that the child needs.

"Cancer Cooties"

In addition to these academic hoops, children who have been diagnosed with a brain tumor face social challenges. Other children may withdraw from them because they have a scary-sounding health problem or fear they might "catch" the brain tumor like a virus.

"Throughout elementary school, I was always afraid of what people would think," one teenager said. "I worried about having no friends. I was shunned by some people who were afraid of getting cancer. The turning point was when I had to give a report in fifth grade—no one laughed and my friends were still my friends."

Another young woman who had a brain tumor as a child recalls that "kids look at you differently." After surgery to remove her astrocytoma, she couldn't go to her ballet class after school; instead, she went to physical and occupational therapy because she had a limp. She also had some cognitive-processing delays that made math difficult for her, so her parents put her into a smaller school that offered extra tutoring with math. Not only did the new school offer her a fresh start socially (because no one knew she had had a brain tumor), but she was able to make a life for herself academically.

Discipline Issues

A mother of a child with a brain tumor says discipline can be tricky. "You don't want the child to be spoiled," she says, "but he already had three strikes against him." It may be difficult to know where to draw the line, but our advice generally is to treat a child with a brain tumor as much as possible as you would treat a child without one.

Teenagers

> *He was two when he was a diagnosed with a brain tumor, so he knows about his experience primarily from our stories. Even so, the yearly MRIs, the concern about the tumor's return, and the shunt between his brain and his abdomen present major extra baggage for a teenager. As far as his tumor goes, his story isn't over yet.*
> —Mother of a brain tumor survivor

Each child's age has its own set of considerations. Even with a brain tumor, kids are still going to be kids and adolescents are still going to do adolescent things. Depending on their child's health, parents have to assess the consequences of a teenager who is driving, with another layer of concern about potential seizures and drug interactions. At this stage, parents may benefit from additional counseling from a professional who is knowledgeable about working with cancer patients. A local chapter of the American Cancer Society can also suggest resources, and a support group through the hospital is helpful at this time.

Teenagers may have the "baggage" of their tumor to carry as they work their way through adolescence. As one girl said, "After how many dates do I say that I have a brain tumor?"

Koocher suggests that parents might look at the teenager's brain tumor experience on a developmental trajectory. As the child is growing physically, intellectually, and socially, what has been interrupted by the illness? How is the brain tumor interfering with the child's normal developmental activities that you would expect him to be involved in at this age? For instance, a toddler who isn't in preschool yet may not know that every child in the neighborhood doesn't have a brain tumor. However, a teenager's primary socialization begins outside the home. He or she will want to look attractive, or look like everybody else, and may be especially self-conscious about appearance at this time. Young women who feel that society expects them to be slim and perfect may be more vulnerable because they may look different or they may fear rejection from peers. The way in which an adolescent manages these issues is often dependent on her personality. Parents should ask themselves, "What is high on my kid's agenda? What is she most worried about and how can I support her in that?"

Teenagers who are struggling with appearance and self-esteem may benefit from "Look good . . . feel better" (www.lookgoodfeelbetter.org), a free, nonmedical program in which cosmetologists offer advice about wigs and makeup. This organization has a program specifically geared to teenagers. Those who have difficulty fitting into a social group at school may need some coaching and support for ways to handle peers and teachers.

Young Adults

As a child, Stacie was always shorter than the other children in her class. When she was nine, she went away to overnight camp for two months, and when she returned her parents noticed that she hadn't grown at all over the summer. They took her to an endocrinologist, who ordered an MRI. It showed a large astrocytoma in her right frontal lobe.

Stacie had surgery to remove the tumor, and now, ten years later, she is doing well. Nevertheless, her parents say that any time she is under the weather, "it freaks us out. Imagine the concerns that parents have for normal kids and magnify that by one thousand."

Stacie's parents didn't give their daughter too much information about her tumor when she was ten, but they realize that as she grows older, she will "someday have to take her health management into her own hands. What if something happened to us?" her father says. "She'll have to advocate for herself."

To guide Stacie toward the independence she will need, her parents have agreed to "let her live her life." It helps that she is a "good kid" who doesn't drink or do drugs; even so, her father says, "We had to let go." Not that letting go has been easy. With Stacie far away in college, her parents worry that she's not getting enough sleep. The fact that she stays up late talking and laughing with her roommates means she's probably not getting enough rest. Even the normal experiences, for which they are grateful, can be cause for concern.

On the college campus where Stacie is studying hotel management, she is mostly private about her health, although her roommates are aware of her history and know what to do if she has a seizure. In general, she and her family have found that "the only people you can really talk with about it are those who walk in your shoes." So her parents are active in a nonprofit organization that supports people with brain tumors and their families. "That's our community," her father says.

Parents can help young adults in this situation by helping to establish a support system wherever they are. Make sure they have connections to doctors in the community and know where the nearest emergency room is located. To prepare the child to manage her own illness, make sure that she knows what symptoms to monitor and whom to call. The child may wear a medic-alert bracelet.

Living with a brain tumor can present concerns at every stage of life, yet today patients have more psychosocial resources and treatment options than ever before. In Part Four, I will describe some of the promising new techniques that are enabling us to succeed in destroying these challenging tumors.

PART FOUR

■

Treatment Options

You are now most likely familiar with the conventional approaches to brain tumor treatment, which include surgery, radiation, and chemotherapy. In the chapters that follow, you will find a guide to these treatment options as well as others with which you may be less familiar. These include "watching and waiting" and newer (novel) therapies that are under clinical investigation. Here you will also find information about drugs for swelling, seizures, and other problems; the forms of supportive care that are available to you should you choose to discontinue treatment; and an overview of treatment options for children with brain tumors.

10

■

Watching and Waiting

One of the most frustrating things about this disease is the feeling of powerlessness. I want to take charge of the situation and respond to the enormous challenge cancer poses but I do not know what to do next.

I am confident that my doctors have given me excellent treatment, but there has to be something I can do beyond taking the medicine and trying to get some exercise.

—Ivan Noble, BBC reporter

It's never over. Every day there is a piece that comes back. You relive part of that diagnosis, part of that surgery. And every time you wait for the MRI results, you wonder if this one is going to be clear.

—Mother of a child with a brain tumor

I know how lucky I am, but you do always think that it's lurking there.

—Long-term survivor of a meningioma

If I run real fast, it won't catch up with me.   —Beau Dyer

Everything you need is inside you.   —Amy Masso

Watching and Waiting
as the First Steps in Treatment

I first met Sandra seven years ago, when she was thirty-five. At that time she had been told she would need surgery immediately to remove a vestibular schwannoma (also called an acoustic neuroma). It was a bad time for her—she had just given birth to her second son, she was in the process of being promoted to the rank of associate professor, and she and her husband were having some marital stress. She came to me in desperation as to whether she could put off surgery to allow her time to get a few things done.

I thought her tumor did not need immediate treatment and that annual MRI scans would be adequate to monitor its growth. Since that time, she has gone on to have a third son, become a professor, and restore peace at home. Her tumor has remained stable.

For some patients, there are several reasons to "watch and wait." Their tumors may not be growing or may progress slowly and not cause symptoms. Colloid cysts, pituitary adenomas, meningiomas, and vestibular schwannomas (acoustic neuromas) may fall into this category. Some older patients and people who have long-term illnesses may have difficulty tolerating some forms of treatment, and the best beginning approach may just be to wait. Finally, some people want to avoid treatment, no matter what, when they are first seen.

If you and your doctors decide to watch and wait as the first step in managing your brain tumor, you will need to consider the relevant signs and symptoms as well as the particular challenges of living with ambiguity. As I mentioned earlier, we can't tell from scans or other tests whether a tumor will grow; and, as you can see from the quotes at the beginning of this chapter, people have different ways of coping with these unknowns.

Watching and Waiting after the Initial Treatment

A second time that watching and waiting may be advisable is after the first set of treatments you receive. Psychologically, this is a different situation than watching and waiting as the first step in treatment. When it is the first step, watching has the implication that nothing is likely to happen. Watching after you have had your first set of treatments may be more fraught with the expectation that a tumor will return. If you are in the "watch and wait" mode, however, it usually means that nothing urgent needs to be done.

Signs and Symptoms to Monitor

If you are waiting and have the same symptoms you had before your diagnosis, don't panic. In many cases, these symptoms do not mean that the tumor is back. Even a seizure can be caused by a delayed irritation of the brain after surgery. Naturally, you should contact your health care team, but don't automatically conclude that this is a sign of recurrence.

If you have any of the following signs or symptoms, however, call your doctor:

- A seizure (often associated with slowly growing tumors)
- Increasing headaches
- Return of previous symptoms—weakness, numbness, speech difficulty, hearing loss, etc.

Usually a simple MRI will establish whether further testing needs to be done or whether everything is fundamentally stable.

Strategies for Coping: Taking It MRI by MRI

We live our whole lives in six-month intervals.

I hate coming to checkups because I'm afraid of bad news. I feel like a dog being dragged to the vet.

We always go as a family. He has his appointment, then we go out to dinner, and then we go our separate ways.

A week before the MRI, it's hard to sleep. I have my scans on Tuesday and don't get the results until Friday. The wait is emotionally draining. Then I get the results and I can be happy for another six months.

I'm superstitious. I always want the same technician, the same scanner.

I'm afraid to ask because I don't really want to hear the answers.
  —Comments by brain tumor patients about watching and waiting

My patients do best if they believe that they'll do well and strive to live as normally as possible. Make life itself the focus of your life, not your tumor. Tell your family and friends that you don't want your illness to be the topic of every conversation.

If you have ever had an infant in the house, you may remember the compulsion to keep checking to make sure that (s)he's still breathing. Most parents don't continue to check on a teenager's breathing several times a night, however—that's not so normal. In the same way, part of moving forward toward wellness while living with a brain tumor involves letting go of some of that vigilance. You will continue to have MRI scans to monitor what's happening in your brain, but you can't allow anxiety and fear to consume you between scans.

What to Expect from Your Regular MRI Scans

Keep up with your scheduled scans. We can do more to treat a tumor successfully if we can see it before you feel it.

If you can, schedule your MRI scan as close to your next appointment to discuss the results as possible. This will help reduce the time you spend worrying and help you preserve your normal routine.

Dr. Malcolm Rogers, a psychiatrist at Brigham and Women's Hospital who has had a long association with our brain tumor group, says that it's not unusual to be very vigilant about symptoms after a brain tumor diagnosis, even with all evidence pointing toward a positive outcome. The everyday aches and pains that all people experience can have a magnified importance, and even a minor headache can seem ominous. You may wish to talk with a mental health professional about handling the stress of wondering if you are really okay.

Integrative therapies such as acupuncture, reiki, prayer, and meditation (see chapter 18) also can help when you are in the waiting mode. As in William Butler Yeats's "The Lake Isle of Innisfree," some people find their own Innisfree—a place, either literal or spiritual, where they can be at peace in the midst of their concern:

> I will arise and go now, and go to Innisfree,
> And a small cabin build there, of clay and wattles made,
> Nine bean-rows will I have there, a hive for the honey-bee;
> And live alone in the bee-loud glade.
>
> And I shall have some peace there, for peace comes dropping slow,
> Dropping from the veils of the morning to where the cricket sings;
> There midnight's all a glimmer, and noon a purple glow,
> And evening full of the linnet's wings.
>
> I will arise and go now, for always night and day
> I hear lake water lapping with low sounds by the shore;
> While I stand on the roadway, or on the pavements grey,
> I hear it in the deep heart's core.

Life Decisions

Painfully I learned not to mourn the future I might have lost. No one has their future until it becomes their present. I have learned not to think too much about the future.

I have tried to live with fear and not surrender to its quiet, corrosive, spirit-sapping power.

I have learned that even with a disease like mine, incurable but sometimes manageable, there are still times when things are getting better.

Today's happinesses create the momentum for tomorrow.

We have accumulated two years of survival from single days and weeks, all of which drew heavily on our strength and will.

—Ivan Noble, BBC reporter

Julia is a thirty-two-year-old woman who began to have seizures two years ago. One morning she woke up and had difficulty speaking, so her husband rushed her to the emergency room of a hospital nearby.

After several tests and scans, doctors discovered that she had a meningioma. The tumor was removed successfully, but she is terrified that it might come back.

Although Julia's brain tumor appears to be gone, she still faces difficult decisions about how to proceed with her life. Because the hormonal changes of pregnancy can trigger growth in a meningioma, she must decide whether to let go of her lifelong dream of having her own child—and, if so, whether it would be fair to consider adopting a child while she has an uncertain prognosis.

People with brain tumors often struggle with life decisions like Julia's. Should they marry? Travel? Continue to participate in sports they love?

My strong opinion is that you should continue on with life as normally as you can, no matter what kind of tumor you have. If there are things you really want to do and you have a malignant tumor, you should do them while you feel good. If you have a benign tumor, you may be surprised that you are alive and well long after you have done those things.

The Glass Is Half Full

But I hear those words "stable" and "remission" and I feel so relieved I want to sleep for a week. I might even risk the first beer in six months. It is wonderful news. We can start making plans again.

—Ivan Noble, BBC reporter

"So much good has come out of this," says a mother of a teenager who was diagnosed with an astrocytoma at age two. "You deal with what you're dealt, and even though the diagnosis turned our world upside down and we'll never be completely out of the woods, this makes you who you are."

Even though the occurrence of a brain tumor is traumatic, it's not all negative. Psychiatrist Malcolm Rogers notes that after the diagnosis, "people sometimes reflect on things and reprioritize their lives, and that can be pretty useful." He finds that sometimes circumstances are very different in reality than they appear on the surface. "If you tap the average person on the shoulder," he says, "people are wrestling with their family lives, work, and friends anyway. This kind of event has a way of pushing people in one direction or another." For instance, a person who goes through the breakup of a relationship before the discovery of the tumor may have felt stuck and unable to move on. Partly because of an altered perception of time, a tumor has a way of freeing people to move on with their lives.

> when despair for the world grows in me
> and I wake in the night at the least sound
> in fear of what my life and my children's lives may be,
> I go and lie down where the wood drake
> rests in his beauty on the water, and the great heron feeds.
> I come into the peace of wild things
> who do not tax their lives with forethought
> of grief. I come into the presence of still water.
> and I feel above me the day-blind stars
> waiting with their light. For a time
> I rest in the grace of the world, and am free.

—Wendell Berry, "The Peace of Wild Things"

11

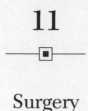

Surgery

People sometimes ask what it's like to be a surgeon who works with the living human brain each day. I think sometimes it's like being Harry Potter—a wizard who has at his command such wonderful technologies as an MRI machine that lets us image the tissue as we remove the tumor, or a global positioning system that lets us navigate through the brain, or an operating microscope that magnifies objects forty times and lets us do very precise surgery. More often, however, it's like Frodo Baggins in *Lord of the Rings*, trying to fulfill a quest against an unknown evil, surrounded by friends and working teams and helped by a little magic. You often feel vulnerable and frightened, despite a brave exterior.

It sounds hokey, but if you are having surgery to remove your brain tumor, your life and that of your surgeon will be intertwined. You will enter into a relationship in which your hopes and concerns are shared. During my career I've learned a lot of things from a lot of people. The people who taught me most, however, are my patients. I've learned how effective advocacy can be from patients who know the literature and challenge their doctors. I've come to admire and respect them.

As you read this chapter, and as you prepare for surgery, consider how important this shared knowledge can be in your quest with your surgeon to destroy your brain tumor. Your surgeon will bring every resource to bear in the operating room, but you can join in the fight by educating yourself about what to expect and by calling attention to symptoms that may signal a complication or a side effect to a drug. With this information, your health care team can help you manage any complications of surgery and exchange a medicine that is causing problems for one that works better for you.

If you or someone you love will have surgery to remove a brain tumor, you will find a brief guide in this chapter. I will try to explain what you need to consider regarding major surgery and will describe the different types of anesthesia, the operation itself, what to watch for during the postoperative period, potential risks and complications, and what we can do to manage them.

Surgery is the first approach for virtually all brain tumors: it establishes the diagnosis and quickly relieves symptoms caused by *mass effect*—the pressure of the tumor on the structures of the brain. Complete surgical removal may cure benign tumors, and we have growing evidence that extensive resection prolongs survival for people who have malignant tumors. There is also compelling evidence that the more completely we remove a tumor, the better the prognosis. This is true for meningiomas, pituitary adenomas, craniopharyngiomas, vestibular schwannomas, pilocytic astrocytomas, and even for medulloblastomas and ependymomas. The trick is knowing precisely where the tumor is; taking it out in a manner that won't hurt the surrounding brain tissue; and being sure it is gone.

Preparing for Planned Surgery

Surgery may be done on an emergency basis after a tumor is found or several weeks in the future, when you have had time to prepare. If you find yourself in the latter situation, here are guidelines to help you get ready for your operation.

Practical Matters: Finances and Paperwork

1. Check your medical, disability, and life insurance policies. Find out if you need to request pre-approval in order for your surgery to be covered by insurance. Identify one contact person through your hospital's business

office (or on your health-care team) who can help you navigate through the maze of co-pays, billing, and deductibles.

2. Make copies of all of these important papers. When you go to the hospital for surgery, take them with you.

3. Ask your doctor where you can find two important documents: a living will and a durable power of attorney for health care.

- A *living will* outlines the kinds of treatment that you would or would not want if you were ever incapacitated and unable to express your wishes about your care.
- A *durable power of attorney for health care (health-care proxy)* names the person you have chosen to make decisions about your medical care for you in the event that you cannot make them yourself. This person might be your spouse, your attorney, or a friend.

Examples of both of these documents are included in the Appendix.

4. Arrange to have your bills paid while you are recovering from surgery. You might establish a payment system through online banking or ask a friend or family member to assume this responsibility.

Preparing Your Colleagues

Outline the requirements of your job for the person who will be stepping in to cover for you at work while you are away. Talk with your employer about when you might be back and what tasks you may be able to accomplish from home until you can return to work. Familiarize yourself with your company's leave policies.

Preparing Your Home

Your children. Will you need to arrange child care? Hire a tutor to help your children with their homework? If they are in school, you may wish to meet with their teachers to discuss ways to support your children while you are away from home and then recovering from surgery.

Food. What about meals? Freeze meals ahead, or ask friends and neighbors who have asked how they can help if they will cover your family's meals for a while. You might ask one person to coordinate the schedule of meals so that your kitchen isn't logjammed one day and bare the next. Some families leave a cooler beside their front door so that friends can leave meals even if no one is home.

Your house. Take care of major household chores now and consider hiring help or asking friends for help with cleaning, maintenance, and yard work. Ask your health care team about what you should expect while you are recuperating at home after surgery. If you won't be able to climb stairs for a while, move your bedroom to the first floor of your house. If you live alone, find out if you should ask a friend to stay with you for a period of time while you regain your strength.

Preparing for Time in the Hospital

When you are packing for the hospital, be sure to include:

Important information:

- Your health insurance card and pre-authorization information from your health insurance company. (Leave copies of this information at home.)
- A list of phone numbers of friends and family members. (Again, leave a list at home or with a friend if you want to appoint him or her as your "chief information officer.")
- A list of every prescription drug you are taking and their dosages.

Creature comforts:

- Travel-size bottles of shampoo, body lotion, and other toiletries. A shower cap.
- Your glasses, dentures, hearing aids, and a watch.
- Soft, comfortable clothing (including a bathrobe) that opens or buttons in front and has wide sleeves.
- Socks and slippers that are not slippery (look for the kind that have treads on the bottom).
- Your own pillowcase.

Pictures, words, and music:

- Movies, books on tape, books, magazines, and a small notebook and pen.
- Copies of photographs of your friends, family, and favorite places.
- A few dollars to pay for newspapers and other items from the hospital gift shop.
- Ask your surgeon if you can bring in a CD to be played during your operation. If a patient asks me to play a specific CD, I and my operating room team will listen to it during the surgery. Some surgeons do not want music to be played because it may distract them, however.

Don't bring: a lot of cash or other valuables (like expensive jewelry) or original documents (unless you have copies).

Good News about Brain Surgery

Advances in surgical techniques and medical imaging mean that brain surgery is much less invasive than it used to be. Many patients report that the operation was less traumatic than they expected—and they are often out of the intensive care unit and back in a regular hospital room after just one night.

Your Preoperative Visit

A few days before your operation, you will go to the hospital where the surgery will take place. This visit may include a physical examination and tests such as:

- Blood tests
- Chest x-ray (if you have not had one in the last five years)
- Electrocardiogram (EKG) (if you are older than 40 or have heart disease)
- Urinalysis

You may wish to donate your own blood in case you need blood during the surgery. This needs to be done several days before surgery.

You will also meet with an anesthesiologist who will explain the type of anesthesia that will be used during your operation. You will be asked to answer questions about your medical history and fill out consent forms and waivers.

Be sure to ask questions about anything that is not clear to you.

Brain Mapping

If your tumor is in or near parts of the brain where motor, language, and other important functions are controlled, your surgeon may want you to have a functional MRI (fMRI) scan before surgery. This type of testing can create a "map" of your brain to help the surgeon determine the best approach to your tumor. This imaging technique, which shows changes in blood flow that correspond to the activity of the brain, can help the neurosurgeon see how different areas of your brain work together. It may allow the surgeon to remove the maximum amount of the tumor while sparing critical areas of your brain.

The Day of the Operation

Customs differ from hospital to hospital. Your health care team will probably ask you not to eat or drink anything after midnight the night before your surgery because vomiting while under anesthesia can be a major problem. They may ask you to shampoo with an antiseptic shampoo. Usually you can take your regular pills with a little water and brush your teeth on the morning of surgery.

When you get to the hospital, you will usually change out of your clothes and put on a hospital gown, and remove your jewelry, contact lenses, and dentures. You will then be given an intravenous line and be attached to instruments that will monitor your blood pressure, heart rate, and blood oxygen level.

At this point your family and friends will go to a waiting area while you are in surgery. In some hospitals, a member of the surgical staff may check in with them intermittently during the surgery. They may be able to take a walkie-talkie or beeper to communicate with the surgical liaison nurse within a one-mile radius of the hospital.

More good news about brain surgery: it's not terribly painful! Most people only require a little acetaminophen for pain relief after a major brain operation. The brain doesn't feel pain.

Drugs You May Given before Surgery

Three types of drugs that you may take before your operation are:

1. *Steroids* to reduce swelling in the brain (often given to patients 12 to 24 hours before a craniotomy).
2. *Anticonvulsants* to control seizures after the operation.
3. *Antibiotics* to prevent infection (just before and up to a day after surgery).

Anesthesia

Different types of anesthesia are used for brain surgery, depending on the location of the brain tumor and the type of procedure.

Intravenous sedation. With this type of sedation, intravenous medications are used to keep you drowsy. This can be an important technique if your tumor is close to the movement or speech areas of your brain, because doctors may need to stimulate those areas during surgery to make sure they're not affected by the procedure. Intravenous sedation allows us to communicate with you while we're doing this because you are not completely "knocked out." Since the brain does not feel pain, this anesthesia is usually well tolerated.

General anesthesia. This is the most common type of anesthesia; with it, you are "put to sleep" with an intravenous injection and anesthesia is maintained with gases inhaled through a tube placed in your trachea (an endotracheal tube).

The Operation

Terms You May Hear

Craniotomy: A surgical opening of the skull in which the bone is taken out and then replaced.

Craniectomy: A craniotomy in which the bone is left out after it has been removed surgically.

Debulking: Surgery to remove as much of the tumor as possible.

Gross resection: Removal of the entire visible tumor.

Lesion: Any abnormality in the brain.

Lobectomy: Removal of one lobe of the brain that may contain the tumor.

Neoplasm: Another name for a tumor.

Resection: Removal of a tumor via surgery.

Partial resection: Removal of part of the tumor.

Radical resection: Removal of the tumor as well as a wide margin surrounding it.

Types of Surgery

One of the first major decisions that patients and physicians face together after the likely diagnosis of a brain tumor is whether to proceed with complete surgical removal of the tumor or whether to have just a biopsy.

For benign tumors, it is usually best to remove the entire tumor if possible, and even for malignant tumors, surgery to remove the tumor has several theoretical advantages over a biopsy. By removing the tumor mass, we can make room to allow for the swelling of the brain tissue that occurs both with radiation therapy and if the tumor recurs. And, obviously, the more tumor we can take out during surgery, the less we will have to treat with other forms of therapy afterward. We can also view the larger mass that we remove during surgery as a bigger and better biopsy sample; our ability to diagnose and grade the tumor is improved because we have more cells to examine. Since the cells often vary throughout a brain tumor mass, and a prognosis is based on the part of the tumor with the highest (most malignant) grade, access to more of the tissue provides us with a clearer picture of the tumor.

The theoretical advantages of surgical removal over biopsy have to be weighed against the added three to four days in the hospital, the potential complications, and the possible longer recovery period after surgery.

Tumor Biopsy

Imaging alone is often inadequate to tell what kind of tumor you have; surgery is usually needed. One of the reasons your doctor may elect surgery is to obtain tissue for a more accurate diagnosis. This procedure is called a biopsy. A biopsy can be done as a small procedure or as the first step in a procedure to remove a tumor.

How Long Will It Take?
A biopsy usually takes from two to four hours.

How Soon Will I Know the Biopsy Results?
After the neurosurgeon obtains a biopsy specimen, it will be sent to a pathologist, who will look at it closely under a microscope to determine what type of cells it contains. Although a preliminary result will be available from the "frozen section" (a laboratory procedure that involves analysis of a frozen slice of the tumor) at the time of surgery, it is usually a week before the final results are available. Occasionally (about 5 percent of the time), the pathologist will not be able to formulate a definite conclusion about the type of tumor based on the sample that he or she sees. In this case, the biopsy is said to be non-diagnostic. In 10 to 12 percent of cases, the diagnosis resulting from the biopsy is unexpected. Instead of a tumor, the sample of cells may suggest another problem, ranging from inflammation to degenerative disease.

How Does a Biopsy Work?
In a biopsy, the surgeon takes a fragment of tumor for examination. There are four ways of carrying out a biopsy. It can be done as part of a craniotomy; with a frame-based system in which a frame is attached to the patient's head (to allow precise targeting of the lesion); with image-guided

techniques involving frameless stereotaxis; and finally, with an intraoperative MR system. Following are descriptions of each:

1. **Craniotomy (open) biopsy.** During an open biopsy, a tissue sample is removed from the tumor after the neurosurgeon has cut a 2- to 4-centimeter hole in the bone and takes tissue directly. This is essentially a craniotomy (see below) for biopsy, but no attempt is made to take all of the tumor out.

2. **Stereotactic (closed) biopsy with a frame.** Your neurosurgeon may perform a stereotactic biopsy if your tumor is very small or located in a deep part of the brain that is hard to reach. Stereotactic surgery, which uses three-dimensional coordinates and CT or MRI to locate a brain tumor precisely, allows us to obtain a biopsy specimen of virtually any abnormality seen on imaging studies.

This procedure may be done with intravenous sedation anesthesia or with general anesthesia. First, a frame is clamped on the patient's head and he or she has a CT or an MRI scan to locate the lesion. The patient is then moved to the operating room, where part of his or her head will be shaved and prepared for the biopsy procedure.

Generally, a small incision will be made in the skin and a hole the size of a dime (a burr hole) will be made in the skull. Then a tiny, hollow probe will be inserted into the tumor and the tumor cells will be drawn up into the probe from an opening in its side. If necessary, biopsy samples can be taken from more than one site during this procedure.

After the biopsy sample has been removed, the needle is taken out and the skin is sewn up. The head clamp is removed. The patient may be admitted to the hospital overnight for observation and will most likely be discharged the next day.

3. **Stereotactic (closed) biopsy with no frame (frameless image-guided biopsy).** As we have been learning to image the brain and navigate with these images, surgeons are now able to do biopsies without a frame attached to the patient's head. For these biopsies, we use a navigation system to display a lesion and then target it. The patient's head must be held still. These systems might be slightly less accurate than the

stereotactic systems that use frames because the reference points are not as fixed.

4. **Intraoperative MR system/stereotactic biopsy in an MRI scanner.** Some institutions, including ours, have a surgical suite with a specially designed magnetic resonance (MR) scanner. This setup allows the surgeon to see MR images during the surgical procedure.

At our hospital, the patient is brought to the scanner and positioned; no frame is required because the scanner acts as the frame. The procedure can be done with a local or general anesthetic—local anesthesia is used if the tumor is in a delicate place. A small area of skin is shaved, prepared, and draped, and local anesthetic is injected. Again, a small opening is made; images are obtained throughout the biopsy to be sure the precise area desired is biopsied. The procedure takes a little longer than conventional biopsies, but it gives the assurance that the target (the tumor) has been reached safely without complication.

Complications of Biopsies

Significant complications of biopsies of brain tumors are uncommon. There is a small risk, about 1 percent, of bleeding, and there is a similar risk of infection. Swelling that can sometimes occur in a malignant tumor can make the neurosurgical difficulties worse. Probably the major risk is that diagnostic tissue is not obtained, but this risk is small depending on the site and size of the tumor (about 5 percent for traditional stereotactic biopsies and 2 percent for biopsies in an MRI scanner).

Standard Craniotomy including Surgery using an Operating Microscope

A craniotomy is the most generally used procedure in brain tumor surgery. It involves removing a piece of the skull and later replacing it.

Preparation. While you are asleep under anesthesia, your head may be placed into a frame to hold it very still during the operation. Usually part of your scalp will be shaved, wiped with an antiseptic solution, and then draped.

Accessing the tumor. Next, the neurosurgeon will make an incision to get to the tumor. He turns back a piece of scalp to expose the bone and then removes it. He exposes the dura, a tough membrane over the brain, and opens it.

Once the brain is exposed, the surgeon can see whether the tumor is lying on its surface or if it might be near the surface, creating a swollen or distorted area. If the surgeon cannot see the tumor, he may use a hand-held ultrasound probe to find it. As he works, he cauterizes blood vessels to control bleeding and gently retracts the brain surface until he sees the tumor.

For tumors in delicate places such as the skull base, the ventricles, or the pineal region, the surgeon will often use the operating microscope to magnify the structures around the region to be operated on. This allows greater precision than would otherwise be possible.

Removing the tumor. Early in the procedure, the surgeon will remove a sample of the mass and give it to a pathologist, who will evaluate the tissue sample by creating a frozen section (he will first freeze it and then cut it into small slices that can be viewed under a microscope). This analysis helps make the diagnosis, but it is only a preliminary one. As the operation progresses, the neurosurgeon will obtain additional samples for "permanent section": these samples are used to make a definitive diagnosis—they will be fixed in formalin (a solution of formaldehyde in water) and stained with more permanent stains.

Often the surgeon can distinguish the tumor from the surrounding brain tissue by the texture, color, and vascularity (blood supply) of the mass. He or she will usually try to remove as much of the tumor as he or she can see, except when it appears to involve a part of the brain that controls movement, speech, or other vital functions. Tumors are usually soft and can be removed with suction or an ultrasonic aspirator, which uses high-frequency sound waves to break up the tumor. The aspirator then sucks up the small fragments.

Closure. The surgeon will close up the covering of the brain (the dura) so that the closure is watertight. Usually the bone will be put back exactly where it was; the surgeon will usually secure it in place with a suture or titanium bands and screws. Less often, if the tumor has invaded the bone and the neurosurgeon cannot put that part of the skull back, another type of mesh or sterile plastic (*cranioplasty*) material is used to cover the opening. Last, the surgeon will close the scalp with staples or stitches. The incision heals in 7 to 10 days.

Image-Guided Craniotomy

Stereotactic technology can be used to guide the surgeon to a chosen target (the tumor) with millimeter accuracy during a craniotomy. With this method, he or she can locate and remove even small, deep-seated tumors with minimal disruption of the surrounding normal brain tissue. This can be done with frameless image guidance or with a stereotactic frame.

This technique is beneficial because it localizes the tumor, so the operation is shorter and the area of the head that the surgeon must disrupt to reach the tumor is often smaller. We can perform this procedure either with general anesthesia or IV sedation.

The initial steps of the procedure (placement of the patient's head in a frame, imaging, and selection of the target tumor and calculation of its exact coordinates) are identical to those for biopsy. The surgeon uses image-guided navigation to determine the location of the bone flap and the tumor.

Craniotomy in a Magnetic Resonance Scanner

The latest imaging techniques are enabling neurosurgeons to do less invasive surgery, even in the most delicate and inaccessible areas of the brain. Sometimes it is difficult for the surgeon to distinguish the tumor from the brain tissue surrounding it. It may also be challenging to completely remove tumors that involve the deep white matter or those that are located in delicate areas—near a ventricle, basal ganglia, or thalamus. In these cases, we have found the magnetic resonance (MR) surgical suite to be invaluable.

The intraoperative MR device at the Brigham and Women's Hospital consists of two doughnut-shaped magnets. The surgeon works between the magnets in the open space that has been draped to become an operative field. Because the magnets can be used for imaging at any time during the operation, we can see real-time images of the brain as we are operating. The MR surgical suite allows rapid reassessment of the removal at any point during the surgical procedure. We can obtain images of the brain at the beginning of the operation to allow for a small, well-placed craniotomy. Once we have removed the bone and opened the dura, we can locate the tumor precisely. We can monitor the extent of resection with periodic images in the middle of the procedure and at the very end, to ensure that we have completely removed the tumor. We can look at one last set of images just after we have closed up the incision to make sure there is no bleeding in the brain.

As with stereotactic craniotomies, we can perform a craniotomy in the MR surgical suite with either IV sedation or general anesthesia. The peace of mind for the surgeon and the patient in knowing at the time of the procedure that the resection is completed without complication is an added benefit.

"Awake" Craniotomy

Tumors sometimes abut or involve a delicate area (such as the functional cortex or subcortical white matter) of the brain so that it may be difficult to completely remove them without causing a new, debilitating neurological problem. One way in which we can overcome this difficulty is to perform the craniotomy with intravenous sedation and intraoperative brain mapping.

If this is the approach your neurosurgeon takes to remove the tumor, you will lie in a comfortable position on an operating table, your head in a frame to hold it still for the procedure. A local anesthetic will be applied to your scalp; during the early parts of the operation and the closure, the anesthesiologist will give you intravenous sedation to make you sleepy.

The reason we don't "put you under" for this type of procedure is that we want you to talk with us and perform "cortical mapping" during some critical parts of the surgery. We use a special type of probe that stimulates the surface of the brain's cortex. As we probe, we can identify areas of the brain that are associated with movement, sensation, naming, and reading. Once we have this information, we may be able to remove all or most of the tumor without causing harm to these sensitive areas. Awake craniotomy in conjunction with intraoperative imaging greatly facilitates our goal of extensive or complete tumor resection with minimal risk to the normal functioning brain.

Local Therapies

Occasionally a surgeon will leave some material in the tumor area to give further treatment after the tumor is removed. For example, Gliadel, a polymer wafer implant soaked with a chemotherapy drug called BCNU, gradually dissolves after several days. This therapy adds some survival advantage to radiation without BCNU, but it is also associated with a slightly higher incidence of infection and swelling.

In some centers, brachytherapy, the implantation of radioactive seeds in the tumor bed, may be used to destroy the tumor "from the inside out." In most centers it has been replaced by radiosurgery, which makes it possible for us to plan the radiation dose more accurately.

Lasers in Brain Tumor Surgery

Sometimes lasers can help to remove a brain tumor, but they require opening the skull; thus they are used during a craniotomy. The carbon dioxide laser, which coagulates only small blood vessels, is the most commonly used tool; it vaporizes tissue without directly touching it. The contact Nd: YAG laser destroys the tissue it touches and also coagulates blood vessels—it can be very useful in destroying a firm, bloody tumor, such as some meningiomas. It can also be used in the intraoperative MRI to destroy a tumor by heating it without doing an open craniotomy.

The Postoperative Period

Congratulations! You have come through surgery safely. Your tumor, or most of it, is gone. Right after your operation, you will wake up and rest for a while in a post-anesthesia care unit (PACU) or other recovery area, or you may be taken directly to an intensive care unit (ICU). Usually patients remain in the ICU for at least 24 hours before they are moved to a regular hospital room, where they may stay from three to five days or more.

Hospital Visitors

You should call your family, especially your children, as soon as possible after your operation. Your voice will be very reassuring to them. Children who are younger than thirteen should not visit you in the hospital. Not only will the environment frighten them, but there is nothing for a short person with a short attention span to do in a hospital setting. They are better off at home with a trusted favorite relative or friend who will not overdiscipline them at this time. Their routines should be kept as normal as possible.

If they absolutely must visit you in the hospital, ask whoever is accompanying them to keep the visit short—no more than 10 minutes—and to stop for ice cream or another treat on the way home.

During your stay in the ICU, monitors will measure your heart rate, blood pressure, and oxygenation. You will probably have a catheter in your bladder, an IV line, a line to measure your blood pressure, and an oxygen mask. You may have pneumatic compression boots to prevent blood clots in your legs.

An experienced team of nurses will observe you carefully. During the first 12 hours after surgery, they will regularly check your heart rate, blood pressure, respiration, the incision, alertness level, and other neurological details. At first you will not be able to ingest anything by mouth except ice chips because anesthesia may leave you feeling nauseated.

Depending on the type of procedure you had, after surgery you may be given medications to:

- Control swelling in the brain (steroids)
- Prevent infection (antibiotics)
- Control seizures (anticonvulsants)
- Control blood pressure (antihypertensives)
- Control pain (usually mild analgesics such as acetaminophen)
- Help your bowels get back to normal
- Prevent blood clots (usually heparin)
- Control fever (antipyretics)
- Control stomach discomfort (antacids) and nausea (antiemetics).

You will be encouraged to get out of bed and sit in a chair as soon as possible after the first day in the ICU. Even this amount of activity can be exhausting after major surgery, so take it slow and listen to what your body is telling you. Remember to keep your doctor informed about how you're feeling.

Potential Risks and Complications

Tumor surgery today is safer than it has ever been. There can be complications, however, and it is important to know what they are. For most brain tumor operations I cite the rate of complications at 5 to 8 percent—that is, there is a 92 to 95 percent chance that everything will go smoothly.

To be thorough, I will list a number of the problems we sometimes find after brain tumor surgery. You should not think any of them will happen to you, however; most are very unusual. They fall into three categories: general medical problems, problems that can occur with any surgery, and problems that are related to the particular surgery you had and the part of the brain affected.

General Medical Problems

Like any surgery, brain tumor surgery can be associated with lung, heart, bladder, or skin problems.

Lung Problems

Atelectasis. Atelectasis is probably the most common problem after brain surgery; it is a blockage of some parts of the lung from secretions that built up while you were in bed for 24 hours. Moisture given by face mask and chest physiotherapy are important steps to prevent it, and neurosurgical ICU nurses can expertly provide these.

Pneumonia. People who have had brain surgery occasionally develop pneumonia, usually 2 to 5 days after the operation. We can treat this condition with antibiotics and chest physiotherapy. Sometimes pneumonia leads to a collection of fluid around the lung, a pleural effusion, that requires drainage.

Deep venous thrombosis and pulmonary embolism. *Deep venous thrombosis* (a blood clot in a vein) sometimes leads to an embolism (blockage of a pulmonary artery) after brain surgery because the clot travels from the vein to the lung. To prevent this problem, you may wear compression stockings on your legs while you are on bed rest. You may also be given injections of heparin, a drug that stops blood clotting in the abdominal wall to prevent this complication.

Pneumothorax. This is a condition in which air enters the space around the lungs; it may require emergency drainage.

Heart Problems

Myocardial infarction. This blockage in the heart arteries rarely occurs after neurosurgery. It is diagnosed by an electrocardiogram (EKG) and by evidence of troponin enzymes in the blood. Tell your health care team right away if you are experiencing chest pain or difficulty breathing.

Cardiac arrhythmias. Irregular heart rhythms can occur, especially in the first few days after surgery. Your nurses will be monitoring your heartbeat carefully.

Bladder Problems

A bladder infection may occur because of the catheter in your bladder. It shows up with irritation on urination after the catheter has been removed. In elderly men, urinary retention may occur because of an enlarged prostate. Because of this condition, some men may need to have a catheter reinserted.

Skin Problems

You may develop a rash from one of the medicines you are taking (especially Dilantin, or a penicillin derivative). This rash can usually be alleviated by stopping the drug. Steroids can produce acne, especially over the shoulders and chest.

General Post-Surgical Problems

A number of problems can occur with any surgical procedure, including brain surgery.

Bleeding

Bleeding in the brain after surgery occurs about 1 percent of the time. It may require further surgery to correct it, although sometimes we can just let the body take care of itself. Increasing headache, a seizure, vomiting that continues to worsen, increasing sleepiness, and weakness on one side of the body may all be signs of a brain hemorrhage, which can be detected by a CT scan.

Infection

An infection can occur in several places after surgery: in the brain itself (an abscess), in the spinal fluid, or in the incision. Infection usually does not occur for a week or more after an operation. A suspected infection in the brain usually requires further surgery to diagnose and drain. A cerebrospinal fluid (CSF) infection is treated with antibiotics—there is also a condition called aseptic meningitis that mimics an infection of the CSF but has no bacteria. An infection in the incision requires opening and drainage and may require removal of the bone. If the wound on your head becomes red, tender, or swollen, or if you develop a fever, tell your health care team.

Problems Related to Specific Locations or Types of Brain Tumor Surgery

Cerebral Swelling (Edema)

When you twist your ankle, you get a lot of swelling for a few days after the injury; it builds up over two or three days. The same phenomenon occurs with surgery for some tumors, especially gliomas and metastases, and especially in tumors of the cerebral hemispheres. The brain around the tumor gets waterlogged and swells. If the area is important for speaking or movement, this swelling may cause delayed worsening in these functions. Generally the swelling improves after five or six days—the best idea of what you will be like a week after the surgery is what you are like immediately after the procedure.

Corticosteroids are given in a high dosage immediately after surgery to help control swelling. They can sometimes mask signs and symptoms of other complications, however. A patient who develops an infection may not have a fever or a stiff neck if he or she is taking this type of drug.

Stroke

Some brain tumors are closely associated with blood vessels, and removing the tumor may lead to a stroke because a blood vessel is blocked during the surgery.

Hydrocephalus

Hydrocephalus is an increase in fluid in the ventricles of the brain. In the first few days after surgery in or around the ventricular system, it can build up quickly because the surgery interferes with spinal fluid absorption. Symptoms include nausea, sleepiness, headache, and vomiting. Usually this needs to be treated quickly because the pressure buildup can be life-threatening.

Over several weeks after any brain surgery, fluid may build up more slowly, producing a condition called "normal pressure hydrocephalus." Key fibers of the brain that are associated with bladder function, walking, and memory can become stretched. The resulting symptoms are difficulty with walking and loss of recent memory.

We often treat hydrocephalus with a ventriculo-peritoneal (VP) shunt, a subcutaneous (under the skin) catheter that runs from the brain to the abdomen to drain away extra fluid. The excess CSF is drained into the peritoneal space of the abdomen (not the stomach!). Shunt valves vary in type—the most sophisticated is a variable pressure valve (the Codman-Hakim valve or the Orbis-Sigma valve) that can be closely adjusted to give optimal results. It can be reset noninvasively, that is, without surgery.

Like plumbing, shunt tubes sometimes clog; signs of shunt malfunction include headache and nausea. They may also get infected; this can only be diagnosed by obtaining a sample of CSF from them.

Cerebrospinal Fluid Leak

Sometimes CSF can leak from bony or other openings after surgery. This needs to be corrected because of the danger of infection. A CSF leak also may be associated with pneumocephalus, or air in the head; it occurs because of a leak that allows CSF out and air in. A CT scan will diagnose this problem; the treatment is usually surgical closure of the leak or a lumbar drain to lower CSF pressure.

Going Home

You may be able to go home as soon as two days after your operation. Sometimes, though, patients need to spend more time in the hospital or in a rehabilitation center for physical, occupational, and/or speech therapy.

Tell your family as soon as you know when you will be coming home so they can prepare. The nurses and doctors will explain your medications and danger signs to watch for before you're released. It is helpful to have someone on hand to take notes.

Once you are home, if you are agitated or cannot sleep at night, you may wish to have one family member spend the night with you and let other family members sleep in another part of the house, or even at a neighbor's house, so that they can get a good night's rest. Give your husband or wife "permission" to sleep elsewhere for a few nights. He or she may feel guilty about asking.

Regardless of when you go home, don't expect too much of yourself too soon. From instant pudding to instant messaging, we are all used to getting results quickly. One of the hardest things to prepare for is that you may not get better quickly after brain surgery. Healing is a gradual process. You may not be up to long visits—or visits at all—from well-meaning friends for a while. If a friend offers to help, ask if he or she can get a book on tape or make a tape or CD of music for you—and leave it in your mailbox. Give yourself time to rest. Work back toward your usual routine slowly.

Follow-up Care

You will have regular visits with your health care team at the clinic as well as regular imaging studies to assess how you are responding to treatment and to allow for early detection if the tumor recurs or there is injury to the brain tissue.

Don't Forget to Celebrate

When your operation is behind you, take some time to experience a sense of relief and victory over your vanquished intruder. A few years ago, a young boy in Virginia, who nicknamed his brain tumor Frank (for Frankenstein), celebrated Frank's death after surgery. The child's mother had auctioned "Frank Must Die" bumper stickers on eBay to help pay for his surgery. The child is still doing well.

Now that you know what to expect regarding a biopsy and surgery to remove a brain tumor, let's continue on to chapter 12, where I will tell you about the various forms of radiation therapy that are other options in our treatment arsenal.

12

■

Radiation Therapy

In most cases, surgery is the first step both toward making a diagnosis and deciding on a course of treatment for a patient with a brain tumor. In certain situations, doctors may follow up with radiation, treating the tumor with x-rays to stem the growth of tumor cells. If you've ever had an x-ray or a CT scan, you've experienced radiation. The radiation used in cancer therapy is similarly painless and invisible. The difference between a CT scan and the x-rays you receive for radiation therapy is the amount of radiation involved.

Radiation therapy is used in several situations. The most common is to treat malignant tumors. Even if you have had an operation to remove all visible tumor, the surgeon may recommend "adjuvant" radiation therapy after the surgery to keep hidden cells around the tumor from growing. After a primary malignant brain tumor is removed, for example, some cancerous cells always remain in the brain around the former site of the tumor. Radiation is recommended to destroy these leftover cells, to prevent a recurrence of growth. Some benign tumors such as skull base meningiomas and pituitary adenomas cannot be completely removed

---

Note: Dr. Stephanie Weiss of the Brigham and Women's Hospital radiation oncology service was particularly helpful in providing information for this chapter.

without compromising brain function. If the tumor that is left shows continued growth after surgery, radiation may be recommended to inhibit further growth. Some benign tumors are located in a part of the brain that would make surgery altogether too risky, so radiation is the only option for treatment. And, finally, some selected tumors, such as vestibular schwannomas, are increasingly being treated with radiation. Overall, radiation may help to treat both benign tumors (such as acoustic neuromas, craniopharyngiomas, and pituitary adenomas) and malignant tumors (such as malignant gliomas, medulloblastomas, and metastases).

Post-surgical Radiation

Post-surgical radiation is usually administered once the cranial incision has healed, about two weeks after the operation. The radiation is delivered in small doses, or "fractions." For patients with primary brain tumors (that is, tumors that originate in the brain), a typical treatment program calls for radiation five days a week over 5 to 6 weeks. Treatment usually lasts for 2 to 3 weeks for people with metastatic disease (tumors that have spread to the brain from cancer elsewhere in the body). The overall duration of treatment will be determined by the radiation oncologist, the specialist who will plan and prescribe your radiation.

If radiation is prescribed in lieu of surgery, the timing of the start date will depend on factors such as the type of tumor, the symptoms you have, and the preparation time for the radiation.

How Radiation Therapy Works

Radiation treatments take advantage of the fact that normal healthy tissue can withstand a low to moderate dose of radiation each day. Normal tissue repairs any damage it sees in about eight hours, so that another dose, or fraction, can be delivered safely the next day. Tumor cells lack the necessary mechanisms that healthy cells have to repair this damage efficiently. With accumulating damage to their DNA with each fraction of radiation delivered, eventually the tumor cells cannot reproduce effectively, and they die.

As long as the tumor is unable to divide, it is considered controlled. So when doctors find that the tumor looks "stable" on a follow-up MRI, this is good news. The tumor may still appear, but it has lost the power to divide. If the tumor is not growing and does not cause symptoms, the treatment is considered successful. Because tumor cells die in stages as individual cells fail to divide, the tumor may gradually shrink over many months after treatment, depending on how fast the cells attempt to replicate.

When treating primary brain tumors, your radiation oncologist will try to protect normal tissue by sculpting the beam to include only areas "at risk," that is, areas likely to harbor the tumor. If the tumor is well demarcated and there isn't likely to be any more outside of what we actually can see on an MRI or CT scan, the oncologists can target the tumor alone. In some cases, the entire brain has to be irradiated: this is usually reserved for metastatic tumors.

How Much Radiation Is Used?

As with radiation to other parts of the body, the amount of radiation to a tumor in the brain is limited by how much radiation the normal tissue around it can tolerate. As I mentioned earlier, the dose per fraction is a big determining factor. Even so, there is only so much total dose you can receive at a given site. These limits have been well studied.

While most medicines are measured in grams or milligrams, radiation is measured in a unit called *Gray* (Gy) or *centigray* (cGy). This is a measurement of the amount of energy that a unit of mass is absorbing. The dose delivered per day and the total overall dose will depend on the kind of tumor that is being treated. For instance, patients with gliomas will typically receive an overall total of 5400 cGy to 6000 cGy in daily fractions of 180 cGy to 200 cGy. Patients with metastases (cancer that has spread from elsewhere in the body to the brain) often will be prescribed 250 cGy to 300 cGy per day to a total dose of 3000 cGy to 3750 cGy.

In some circumstances, your doctor will recommend a special kind of boost to fight an obvious tumor; that is, an extra dose of radiation to the lesion itself without inclusion of normal tissue in the prescribed field. In this case, the dose can be five to ten times that normally given in one fraction: this is called *radiosurgery*. If the target is too big for radiosurgery (usually bigger than 3 cm) or near a sensitive structure your doctor is concerned about, he or she may recommend a smaller focused dose per day over several days. This is called *stereotactic radiotherapy*. As I mentioned in the last chapter, stereotactic therapy involves a carefully calculated target.

Specialists You May Meet

- *Radiation oncologist:* This physician is the captain of the radiation treatment team. He or she will plan your care.
- *Dosimetrist:* This specialist, who usually has an engineering or physics background, is an expert at figuring out how to get the radiation to the spot the doctor prescribes. Dosimetrists are like the pharmacists of radiation.
- *Radiation physicist:* This specialist is responsible for assisting with the radiation plan and overseeing the machines that emit radiation.
- *Radiation therapist:* This member of your health care team, who is not a physician, will actually administer your radiation therapy.
- *Radiation oncology nurse:* This nurse will guide you through the treatment process and will be available to answer your questions and help you manage the side effects of radiation therapy.

Radiosensitizers

Sometimes drugs are given during the course of radiation to make radiation more effective. These are *radiosensitizers*. Combined with the radiation, the two together are greater than the sum of their parts and seem to kill tumor cells more effectively. In this case, your radiation oncologist, or a doctor who specializes in administering chemotherapy, either a neuro-oncologist or a medical oncologist, may prescribe the radiosensitizer. Temozolomide (Temodar) is a common radiosensitizer. Other drugs under study include RSR13, the farnesyl transferase inhibitor R115777, the EGFR inhibitor tarseva, gadolinium texaphrin, and TM-601.

Preparing for Radiation Treatment

Your radiation oncologist will be in charge of your radiation treatment. Every week, you will meet with him or her and a nurse for an "on treatment visit" (OTV). During this visit, your radiation team will talk with you about your symptoms, questions, diet issues, pain issues, any lab results, plan of care, and medicines.

During a course of radiation therapy, your nurse most likely will ask you to use only mild, fragrance-free and lotion-free soap. Treat your scalp with mild shampoos: do not use gels, sprays, color, or perms for your hair. Avoid temperature extremes (like ice or heat packs) on your head.

Your skin should be clean and dry before you receive radiation. You can use lotions after your daily treatment to help alleviate any irritation. If you need anything on a day other than the scheduled day to meet with your radiation oncologist, don't hesitate to ask; just ask any member of the treatment team to help.

Although you should feel no different after daily treatment, you should have someone come with you the first day or so, just until you're used to the routine. Ask your doctor about restrictions on driving that may be related to your tumor.

Terms You May Hear

- *Simulation:* The simulation, or "sim," is a mapping procedure that enables your team to figure out how best to arrange the radiation beams in your situation, and how best to protect the normal areas of the brain. Often a mask, much like a fencing or hockey mask, is made at the sim. After all the mapping has been done at the sim, the doctor and the team will want to make sure you're lined up exactly the same way, day to day. The mask will help to accomplish this. Marks may be made on the mask and perhaps on your skin.
- *Margin:* The margin is the area immediately surrounding the tumor in the radiation field. We apply radiation to both the tumor and the margin if we suspect that some tumor cells may spread into the healthy tissue that surrounds it.

- *Conedown:* Often during many weeks of treatment, the radiation oncologist may recommend that the last few treatments focus on only the tumor or tumor bed with a smaller margin around the field. This is called a conedown.
- *Boost:* Another name for a conedown. This may also refer to a single high dose of focused radiation delivered by radiosurgery.
- *Port:* The treatment field where the radiation is focused.

Types of Radiation Therapy

External Beam Radiation Therapy and Brachytherapy

The first distinction in radiation therapy is between external beam radiation and brachytherapy. Most patients who are prescribed radiation receive external beam radiation therapy (EBRT). This is a broad term and refers to any treatment delivered from a machine some distance (usually a few feet) away from you. The alternative is brachytherapy, where radioactive sources are implanted directly in a tumor bed. This is not done as much in the treatment of brain tumors as it is in other cancers, like prostate cancer. (New York's former mayor Rudolph Giuliani publicly discussed his brachytherapy treatment for prostate cancer.)

EBRT can be delivered in many ways and your doctor will talk with you about which form is most appropriate for your needs. The most common types of EBRT are whole-brain radiation, 3D conformal radiation, intensity-modulated radiation therapy, stereotactic radio*surgery,* and stereotactic radio*therapy.* These generally differ in terms of the technique of administration.

With all EBRT, it is important to know that the treatment will not make you radioactive. The radiation is very much akin to a flashlight in that it is a beam that is active only when the machine is switched on. As soon as the beam is off, the radiation is gone. It has done its work for the day at the DNA level. This means that even immediately after your daily treatment, you can be near children, pregnant women, and pets safely, without restriction. The only exception is that women should not be pregnant, or get pregnant, during treatment. The radiation is harmful to a sensitive developing fetus that comes with the mother into the treatment room. You must use precautions to ensure that you do not become pregnant during treatment. If you think you may be pregnant or become so during treatment, *tell your radiation oncologist immediately.*

In radiation therapy, new techniques are evolving all the time. I would encourage you to explore the different types of radiation available, but remember that treatment is dependent on the kind of tumor you have—you may not be a candidate for all of them. Your radiation oncologist can assess your eligibility. Below are some of the more common techniques used in external beam radiotherapy.

Whole-Brain Radiation

Whole-brain radiation is usually delivered if there is concern that there may be small deposits of tumor cells in the brain that are not visible on MRI or CT. Even though other techniques of radiation may target specific lesions, that sort of precision would fail to deal with any microscopic disease that is waiting to grow and could, over time, cause significant symptoms. In the case of metastasis, doctors consider the likelihood that there may be other deposits of cancer cells too small to actually see ("microscopic" disease) elsewhere in the brain. In that case the entire brain is treated.

As scary as this sounds, the process is generally simple and well tolerated. The treatment is usually planned ("simmed"—short for simulated) on a machine much like a typical x-ray machine. At the sim, x-ray films are taken of the left and right side of your head. The radiation oncologist will then draw blocks on these films to block the portions of your anatomy that are to be shielded from the treatment field. This typically includes the area above your eyebrows and across your ears on down.

3D Conformal Radiation

For both benign and malignant tumors, your radiation oncologist may recommend 3D conformal radiation therapy (3DCRT). This sort of treatment is best for patients whose condition requires treatment that extends to a margin (usually a few inches) around the tumor bed to account for microscopic disease. Gliomas are typically treated this way. In this case, the sim generally involves a CT scan done specifically for the sim. This scan becomes the map your doctor uses to plan your treatment. The CT scan will allow your doctor to use an electronic crayon to contour the area she wants to treat and the normal structures she wants to protect (for instance, the nerves to the eyes). She will likely also order an MRI to help with the planning. MRIs often show the anatomy of the brain and tumor better than CT. Usually an MRI is fused (overlaid) onto the CT sim to help direct the contouring.

Using the sim images as a 3D model, the radiation oncologist can figure out how to arrange the beams in three-dimensional space to make the best configuration to treat what she wants to treat and block out what she wants to protect.

It might help if you think about 3D conformal radiation like this: Imagine a flashlight shining on a target. You can see one strong bright beam making a path to the target being illuminated. Now imagine one strong beam going into the body. If the equivalent method were used in radiation therapy, the beam would pass through normal tissue to reach the tumor, exposing those normal areas to a dangerously high dose of radiation in the process. Now suppose instead that we take three or four flashlights, each with beams that are one-third or one-fourth of the intensity of the one strong flashlight. If each of those beams is pointed from a different direction onto the same target, the spot where they converge gives off the *same intensity as one strong beam.* This is exactly how radiation is planned. Though there are many beams (usually three or four), each beam is relatively weak and passes through the normal tissue without much effect. But where they converge over the tumor, the beams add up to enough dosage to kill the tumor cells.

Normal tissue is also protected by blocks that shape the beam and "block it out" over normal tissue. The blocks, which simply keep radiation from reaching certain tissue, may be physical blocks that are placed in the head of the machine. Sometimes they are a part of the machine and made of sliding metal fingers, or "leaves." The leaves can slide all the way in or all the way out of the field as the doctor designs it, or any way in between.

As you can imagine, after all this mapping, your doctor and the therapists who will treat you on the machine want to make sure you are lined up in the correct position every time you receive radiation therapy. Thus, at your simulation session, you'll likely have a special plastic mask made for you to wear during treatment. It looks very much like a fencing or hockey mask and will fit only you. It may be marked to help the therapists line you up in it. You will probably wear this mask for about 5 to 15 minutes each day—the typical duration of each treatment.

You should feel the same coming out of treatment every day, without any increasing fatigue or other symptoms. Later common side effects of treatment include partial hair loss on your scalp where the beams enter, some fatigue, and mild skin irritation that can be soothed with special lotions after daily treatment. Your doctor should review any likely side effects that are particular to your specific diagnosis. I will address side effects in more detail toward the end of this chapter.

Intensity-Modulated Radiation Therapy (IMRT)

Intensity-modulated radiation therapy (IMRT) is a form of three-dimensional conformal radiation therapy (3DCRT) that is appropriate for both benign and malignant tumors. IMRT takes advantage of modern computers and machine technology in helping the doctor protect normal tissues. IMRT uses radiation-blocking leaves to "sculpt" the shape of the dose (usually a concave shape) around sensitive structures. For instance, let's say the doctor is concerned about the dose to the optic nerve that supplies vision to the eye. The computer divides each field into small pixel-like segments. While the beam is on, the doctor can prescribe the dose so that the leaf enters the field for part of the time, thus creating a "cool spot" where needed. This can be done for the beams coming in from several different directions. This is how the intensity of the beam is modulated. IMRT takes longer than the other forms of treatment to deliver (from 15 to 45 minutes per treatment) because of the complexity of the plan. Its side effects are the same as those associated with 3DCRT.

Stereotactic Radiosurgery (SRS)

Some brain tumors are discrete and well encapsulated; these include both benign tumors (acoustic neuromas, pituitary adenomas, meningiomas) and malignant tumors (metastases that are obvious on MRI and CT). Radiosurgery is a good treatment for these tumors.

In radiosurgery, a single high dose of radiation is given to a relatively small tumor, typically less than 3 or 4 cm in greatest dimension. Several machines can deliver radiosurgery. You may hear them referred to by the names Gamma Knife and Cyberknife or hear the terms "linac-based" or "cobalt." They are all ways to perform radiosurgery, much like both Coca-Cola and Pepsi are colas.

There are some key differences among these machines. The *Gamma Knife* uses 203 separate radioactive cobalt sources that all aim at the same target; it is particularly good for small targets. This type of therapy is given after a "radiation source helmet" is placed on the patient's head. The *linac radiosurgery system* uses pizza-like slices of radiation that all converge on the tumor. The beams can mimic the shape of the tumor and conform tightly around it. The *Cyberknife* is a low-energy linear accelerator mounted on a robot that performs radiosurgery; this procedure does not require the placement of a frame fixed to the patient's skull. *Proton beam radiosurgery* uses a particular feature of protons to minimize the radiation given to normal tissue around the tumor.

The terms "radiosurgery" and "Gamma Knife" are misleading. There is no actual invasive surgery involved in this procedure, and no knife. As in conformal radiation and IMRT, many beams will be used, coming in from many directions, and they will converge on a single point: the tumor. But unlike other types of radiation, in radiosurgery the intended port for the treatment is *only the tumor itself.* There is no margin added to include normal tissue that may harbor microscopic disease. Because of this, the beams must be relatively small and "sharp," that is, the radiation dose must fall off very quickly.

Imagine a stone being thrown into a pond. You get a big splash where the stone lands, and where the radiation is aimed. Then you get ripples out from the splash, each ripple farther away and flatter than the one inside it. The radiation dose will fall off in the same way. Where the beam is aimed is like the initial "splash" where the dose is concentrated. This splash is called the "isocenter." As you move away from the isocenter, the intensity of the dose falls off quite precipitously. By the time you're an inch or two away from the edge of the tumor, there is negligible dose left. Your doctor will make sure the radiation is prescribed so that the edge (margin) of the tumor gets enough treatment.

Radiosurgery is generally accomplished in a long one-day procedure that includes mapping simulation, planning, and treatment. Aside from the difference in fractionation (one day versus several weeks), radiosurgery is different from typical external beam radiation in terms of how you are set up on the treatment table. With fractionated radiation, you usually wear a plastic mask that relocates you day after day on the table in treatment position. Since the targeting in radiosurgery must be exact, a frame that allows accurate planning is attached to your head. This is exactly the same frame used in stereotactic surgery.

The procedure is relatively nonintrusive. At our institution the treatment is as follows. The morning of the procedure, a topical anesthetic cream is rubbed in four spots over your forehead and the back of your head. Your neurosurgeon then places a special, halo-like frame on your head for the day using local anesthesia in four spots. During the day you can rest your head back in a comfortable chair with the frame on and you can eat, watch videos, and interact with others normally.

After your frame goes on, you will have a planning scan, either a CT or MRI. This scan may be fused (overlayed) with scans you received prior to the radiosurgery day and will serve as a map for the doctor to locate important structures and arrange the radiation beams around them. The frame that you are wearing during the sim will act as an external reference point to assure that you are in the same exact position for treatment. Radiosurgery is so accurate that when you go to treatment, you will be lined up to within 1 millimeter of the same position you were in during scanning. That is little more than the width of the period at the end of this sentence.

Most people find that the worst part of the day of radiosurgery is the waiting around. Remember, unlike conventional radiation therapy, radiosurgery requires that the simulation, planning, and treatment be done all in one day. After your sim, you will be able to relax, read, sleep, or watch TV. It's a lot like jury duty in that we need you to hang around in the department all day. Bring a video or a book. Cards and puzzles can also help to pass the time. Some facilities will offer you a place to play your music or watch television and DVDs. Often family and friends will be allowed to accompany you for the day—while you're not in treatment, of course.

While you're waiting, your doctor will be working with the dosimetrists and physicists to do the radiation plan. Again, the emphasis will be on contouring the important structures like your normal anatomy (eyes, brain stem, optic nerve) and the tumor. The radiation oncologist will arrange the beams so as to concentrate the dose on the tumor and spare the normal tissue. After a plan has been approved, the physicists will take care to verify the coordinates on the machine and do a "dry run" to assure that you will be set up just as planned. A few hours later, you will be brought to the machine and will lie down on the treatment couch while the radiation is delivered. This typically takes from a half hour to an hour and a half, depending on the number of lesions being treated that day and the complexity of the plan. In fact, most of the time you're on the table, the machine is just lining up properly to deliver the radiation accurately. The time the beam is on is much less.

During the treatment, you will be alone in the room; however, a closed-circuit camera with two-way audio will be on the whole time. This way you and the team can communicate during the entire procedure. The team may come in between "beam on" times to set up the next beam.

When treatment is done, you will be taken back to have the frame removed by the neurosurgeon. This takes only a couple of minutes and is typically painless. You may experience a mild pressure sensation in your head, which usually goes away in about five minutes. The pin sites from the frame—which sometimes leave sore spots and tenderness—will usually heal within a week. Your nurse will give you instructions for keeping your skin clean over the next 24 to 48 hours before you can resume your normal bathing.

For most people, side effects from radiosurgery are minimal or entirely absent. You will likely be sent home with some medications to take for a brief period of time to help minimize any side effects such as headache, nausea, or seizure from treatment-related swelling. Even though you didn't have invasive surgery, radiation does kill tumor cells. This can cause some local swelling in the brain tissue. The medications will make it unlikely that you will have any significant side effects from this temporary swelling. The best part of radiosurgery is that at the end of the day, you get to go home and sleep in your own bed.

Frameless Radiosurgery/SRS (the Cyberknife)

Some radiosurgery systems today are moving to frameless treatment. These include the Cyberknife, which is a linear accelerator mounted on a rotor, and the Trilogy system, which modifies a traditional linear accelerator. The obvious advantage of a frameless system is that it spares you from the whole process of the frame placement and having to wear it all day. Before this system, doctors needed to make sure that the accuracy without a head frame was as good as what we can do with frame-based radiosurgery. Some systems, such as the Cyberknife and Trilogy, have successfully created that precision.

In frameless treatment, cameras, mounted in the treatment room, are dynamically linked to the treatment machine. As you move, the treatment device moves. Fine adjustments can be made while you are on the treatment table, ensuring the same level of accuracy as conventional radiosurgery. The use of "onboard imaging" such as this is why frameless radiosurgery is sometimes called "image-guided." However, not all image-guided procedures are frameless, and as other parts of this chapter have made clear, most radiation nowadays uses exquisite imaging. So for our purposes, we'll call this technique "frameless SRS."

Stereotactic Radiotherapy (SRT)

Sometimes radiosurgery isn't appropriate because the tumor is too big (greater than 3 centimeters) or because it's too close to a sensitive structure like the optic chiasm where the optic nerves meet. Your radiation oncologist can still provide effective radiation to the tumor with stereotactic radiotherapy (SRT). The term "radiosurgery" implies a one-day treatment. In SRT, sometimes called *fractionated stereotactic radiotherapy* or *FSR*, your radiation oncologist will deliver treatment to the lesion, with virtually no surrounding tissue included, over several days or weeks. Because this requires more than one day of treatment, it's not reasonable to use a rigid radiosurgical frame affixed to your head, as in SRS. Instead, a special conformal plastic mask is made at the sim that can be taken off and relocated the next day for treatment. It is similar to the mask used in 3DCRT, but because we don't want a margin this time, it must be set precisely, usually within a couple of millimeters of accuracy each day. Typically this mask will include a piece that goes in your mouth called a "bite-block." This assists with the daily setup.

The mask is made at the time of the sim, which takes about 5 to 10 minutes. It is made of malleable plastic that molds to a shape when it is heated. It is warmed in a hot water bath and cools on your face so it fits only you. Some people describe it as a little like getting a facial or the preparation for a hot shave; others say that it actually hurts for a brief time. If you have any anxiety about wearing the mask, ask your nurse for an anti-anxiety medication prior to treatment. The mask is made in a mesh pattern, again much like a fencing or hockey mask, so you can breathe easily through it.

Proton Beam Radiation Therapy

All of the types of radiation mentioned so far use photon energy. Another form of radiation treatment acts differently, with particles known as protons constituting the radiation beam. Though both methods are invisible and the experience for the patient is essentially the same, they do allow for a crucial difference in outcome.

I compared photons to a flashlight, where the beam creates a pathway through normal tissue to the target. But what happens after the photons hit the target? In fact, there is "exit" radiation beyond. This is a relatively weak dose of radiation, but it is noticeably present. In some cases, there is a need to have the radiation dose fall off to zero after it hits the target. Usually this is because there is a sensitive structure right behind the focal point and the amount of radiation dose needed to control the tumor exceeds the tolerance of this structure. This may be a particular concern in the case of a recurrent tumor, where the radiation given has reached the tolerance limit of the normal tissues. This is also important in the case of the treatment of children, whose normal tissue is still growing, thereby posing a risk of developmental delay due to radiation exposure. Charged particle radiation composed of protons has that unique property wherein the exit dose is nearly negligible. This feature is called "the Bragg peak."

A machine called the Cyclotron delivers protons. It's a very big and very expensive device and there are only a small number currently operational in the United States. Thus, it is used only in selected cases. Remember, too, that sometimes we want the field around the tumor treated for microscopic disease. We have had good results with proton beam therapy in the treatment of skull base chondrosarcomas and chordomas, as well as melanoma of the eye and medulloblastomas.

When we talk about protons, we are only describing the type of radiation being used, but nothing about the technique. Protons can be delivered as conformal therapy and as radiosurgery.

Other Types of Radiation Delivery Devices

Boron Neutron Capture Therapy. A few other ways to receive radiation are limited in their use. Boron neutron capture therapy (BNCT) involves an intravenous injection of a stable boron-10 compound. Tumor cells absorb this more than normal brain cells. The radiation is delivered with another form of radiation called thermal neutrons. When the neutrons hit the boron-containing tumor, the boron becomes an unstable boron-11 and gives off another set of high-energy alpha particles. The alpha particles are heavy and travel only about one cell length. They deposit a lot of energy in the boron-containing tumor and kill the tumor cells.

This technique requires the boron to be taken up much more in tunor cells than in normal brain cells. Scientists are currently working to create boron compounds that will better concentrate in tumor cells.

Heavy Particle Radiation Therapy. Helium and neon are two heavy particles that can damage DNA. Essentially, these particles seem to deposit more "dose" per unit of radiation than do photons. They are thought to possibly be superior for "radioresistant" tumors, which are tumors that normally do not respond to radiation. Of course, the trade-off may be more damage to the normal tissue. Heavy particles are in limited use in the United States.

Neutrons. Neutrons are particles that have no charge (they're "neutral"). They do their damage through a different mechanism in the DNA than photons or charged particles. They are more commonly recommended in head and neck tumors and have not yet been used widely for brain tumors.

Experimental Radiation Therapies. Experimental forms of radiation therapy are always under way. Antiprotons are being investigated to see if they might be used in the clinic. They would work like protons but also create an "annihilation" reaction at the end of their path. This would actually release additional protons and create more damage in the tumor. Pion therapy works in a manner similar to protons.

While Being Treated with Radiation . . .

In general, you can eat anything you want while you are undergoing conformal radiation therapy. Stay well hydrated and don't try to lose weight at this time. Good nutrition is important. If your appetite is off, talk with your nurse about high-calorie, high-protein supplements that can help you maintain your weight. Try eating smaller meals throughout the day rather than three larger meals. Lean protein, fruits, vegetables, complex carbohydrates, and some fats are all important parts of your diet now, as always.

You should talk to your doctor about any supplements you may be taking. They may interfere with the radiation or any chemotherapy or radiosensitizers you are receiving. In particular, because radiation works by oxidation, high doses of anti-oxidants such as vitamins C, A, and E and co-enzyme Q (CoQ10) and lycopene can make radiation treatments less effective. You may take a multivitamin if it does not include more than 100 percent USRDA of these anti-oxidants. Tell your health-care team if you are taking any vitamins, supplements, or pain relievers.

For more information about different types of radiation therapy for adults with brain tumors, contact the Radiation Therapy Oncology Group (RTOG), www.rtog.org, a clinical cooperative group funded by the National Cancer Institute.

Side Effects of Radiation Therapy

To most people, Joan would seem very lucky. She had an anaplastic astrocytoma in the left temporal lobe removed eight years ago. After her surgery, she had radiation therapy. Yet now, at the age of forty-two, she feels that she is not very lucky. Her memory is bad, she is having trouble thinking of the names of things, and she is perpetually tired. She is an example of someone who would not have survived a generation ago, but now that she has survived she is dealing with long-term challenges that are, at least in part, a result of her radiation treatment.

Short-Term Side Effects

Fatigue
Fatigue is a common side effect of any radiation therapy. It usually starts somewhere in the middle of your treatments and it may be several weeks before you're feeling back to normal with regard to energy. Some of this is dependent on your overall health prior to and during treatment.

Honor the fatigue by allowing yourself to rest. "Fighting through it" doesn't help. But don't become a couch potato. Short naps (less than an hour) will give you a boost without making it difficult to sleep at night. If possible, try not to deviate from your usual sleep routine.

Stay as active as you can be while remaining comfortable. Activity can help prevent you from becoming deconditioned. Walking and gentle exercise (yoga, swimming, or t'ai chi) may help. Even daily short walks can help prevent blood clots from forming in your legs. If you notice any pain, redness, or swelling in your legs, let your doctor know *immediately*. These may be symptoms of blood clots. If a blood clot breaks off, it can go to the lungs—a potentially fatal event. Make sure to consult with your radiation oncologist and neurosurgeon to see if they have any specific restrictions for you.

Work back to your usual level of activity gradually. Don't try to do more than you are ready to do. If you are struggling with severe or prolonged fatigue, your health-care team may prescribe medication like Ritalin or Provigil to help boost your energy level.

Brain Swelling

Any treatment to tissue can cause inflammation and swelling. If you had surgery, you were probably taking steroids for a short time to prevent swelling. Swelling can occur during radiation as well. This may cause a flare-up of the symptoms you experienced prior to diagnosis of your tumor. If so, let your radiation oncologist or nurse know. They can assess if this is just a little swelling that can be relieved with medication or if it is something they want to investigate further. Sometimes swelling can cause a headache or nausea even if you never had these symptoms before. Most patients don't have a problem with this, and it virtually always can be controlled. Severe headache or nausea is never normal. Contact your team or on-call doctor immediately if you experience these or any symptoms that are new for you.

Skin Irritation

Your scalp may become temporarily irritated, itchy, or reddened because of radiation therapy. While you are going through radiation therapy, use only warm water and a mild soap and baby shampoo. Don't use soaps that contain deodorant or any aluminum products, perfumes, makeup, powder, or aftershave. Talk with your nurse about the skin products you use.

If your skin is itchy and dry, moisturize it with a gentle product. Ask your nurse what he or she would recommend. Remember to apply moisturizers *after* your radiation treatment—not before.

When you wash your face and hair, be gentle. Don't rub them dry with a towel. Likewise, save a massage to reward yourself *after* your skin has had a chance to regroup from radiation therapy—not before.

Avoid extreme, direct temperature changes to your skin due to hair dryers, heating pads, and ice packs. Bathe or shower with lukewarm water. Also, stay away from hot tubs, saunas, and direct sun. Wear a soft hat when you go outside and use sun block (SPF 15 or higher) all over your exposed skin if you do go out. You will need to be especially vigilant about sun protection for many months after your radiation therapy ends.

Many people find that a few weeks after the therapy is over, their skin gets back to normal and they can begin to use the type of soap, shampoo, and lotions that they used before radiation therapy began.

Ear Congestion

Another side effect of radiation therapy is congestion in the ears—a feeling you may recognize if you travel much by plane or ever got water in your ears after swimming. This feeling dissipates as gradually as it occurs, usually a few weeks after treatment ends.

Ear drops can help to ease this discomfort. Tell your health-care team if you have difficulty hearing or if there is drainage from your ear.

Hair Loss

Alopecia, or hair loss, can happen during or immediately after radiation therapy for the same reason it can occur after chemotherapy—both stop fast-growing cells from dividing effectively. Unless you are having whole brain radiation, you will probably only lose hair on the part of your head where you received radiation, so you may have a spotty hairdo to contend with. You will not lose hair on your face or body. Typically hair loss begins 2 to 4 weeks into treatment (depending on the size of the daily dose and the sum total dose). It tends to start rather suddenly, one morning while brushing your hair or in the shower. Often people suddenly notice hair on their pillow. Your physician can advise you about what to expect ahead of time.

Hair loss from treatment is upsetting because your hair is a major part of your self-image and identity. Hair loss from radiation isn't voluntary like a haircut, and it's a reminder of what you're going through. It's completely normal to be sad and angry about hair loss.

After whole-brain irradiation, it may take up to two years for your hair to grow back. After focal radiation (radiation that is limited to a specific area), your hair may grow back sooner, within four to six months. If you are taking chemotherapy while undergoing radiation therapy, it may take longer. The extent to which hair grows back is partially dependent on what other treatments you've had. People who have had a lot of chemotherapy often find it never fully grows back as it was. Hair growth after radiation is very different from the growth right after a haircut because right after you get a haircut the follicles start growing right away. After radiation or chemotherapy, it takes longer. Also, when your hair returns, it may have a different color or texture than before, and it may be thinner on the top of your head.

If you think you may want a wig at some point, see a wigmaker before you begin radiation therapy. Most wigmakers like to see the way you like to wear your hair. Your doctor can write you a prescription for a wig and your health insurance may cover it. Talk with the wigmaker to make sure that the lining of the wig does not irritate your scalp.

Depression

Although frequent visits to the hospital for treatment can be physically and emotionally draining, once your radiation therapy is over, you may find that your regular visits were reassuring. You may have felt, at least, that you were doing something to fight your tumor. Some people find it hard to move ahead without consistent appointments.

If you are feeling anxious and depressed, talk with your health care team about how to find a support group. Many hospitals also have social workers, psychologists, psychiatrists, and religious counselors who can help you through this difficult time. See chapter 18 for more information about support groups.

Eye Irritation

If your eyes feel irritated or dry after radiation therapy, warm water compresses and eye drops may help. This side effect usually goes away a few weeks after radiation therapy ends.

Long-Term Side Effects of Radiation Therapy

"Late effects on normal tissue" are the long-term side effects of radiation therapy. They may include mild to moderate difficulty with short-term memory; hormone imbalances; and non-symptomatic damage to the good brain tissue around the tumor (called radionecrosis) seen on post-treatment scanning. More severe long-term symptoms and symptomatic radionecrosis are relatively uncommon. Rarely, radiation can induce the development of a secondary tumor. These rare tumors, when they occur, may be either benign or malignant and tend to occur many years after treatment.

Radiation Necrosis

After your radiation treatments are over, your oncologist will schedule appointments for you to have MRI or CT scans. Sometimes these scans show an effect of radiation on normal tissue called "white matter changes" or "radionecrosis." These changes can occur many months or even years after your radiation therapy is over. Typically, radiation changes are asymptomatic and only notable on scans. Occasionally people experience symptoms with radiation necrosis. These symptoms can resemble those of a brain tumor and reflect the region of the brain that is being disturbed: they include problems with vision, coordination, and headache. Sometimes we can't tell necrosis from recurrent disease on routine MRI or CT scans. Some metabolic imaging such as PET scans or MRI spectroscopy can help differentiate the two and surgery can tell definitively what is going on and relieve symptoms.

A New Tumor

Rarely, several years after radiation therapy, another tumor can develop in the part of the brain that received radiation. This new tumor probably results from mutating damage to the DNA of normal brain tissue and blood vessels. Such a lesion may be either benign or malignant. If the lesion is found incidentally on routine follow-up and its appearance is consistent with a benign lesion such as low-grade meningioma, this may be followed with serial scanning. Sometimes the tumor will require surgery for diagnosis and symptom relief. The overall plan will depend on the findings during the workup.

Regular follow-up MRI and CT scans can help to identify secondary tumors—and they can also reveal good news, that the radiation treatments have shrunk the treated tumor and spared the surrounding brain tissue from necrosis.

Difficulty with Memory

Sometimes radiation therapy can lead to difficulty with short-term memory. Typically, you might note that several months after radiation, you are more inclined to make lists before going shopping, or that you need to make a note of where the car is parked in an unfamiliar garage. You might find that you misplace your keys a little more than usual. The people most at risk for these side effects are people who already have an underlying process of small-vessel disease. This typically includes people with high blood pressure, high cholesterol, heart or blood vessel disease, and diabetes. More severe side effects are uncommon.

If you are working through these issues after radiation therapy, let someone on your health care team know. Behavioral neuropsychiatric testing can identify where the problem areas lie and your health care provider can help you find ways to fix or accommodate them.

Hormonal Insufficiency

If your pituitary gland, the gland that secretes several key hormones, was in the radiation field, your thyroid hormone, or other hormone, levels may be off. This condition is typically easily remedied by a thyroid hormone replacement pill or other hormone replacement. You should go for regular checkups for many years to be sure there is no loss of pituitary function.

Radiation therapy can be one of the most important tools for controlling brain tumors. For malignant tumors, it significantly adds to survival, and for metastases, stereotactic radiosurgery has become one of the most important techniques we have for definitive management. For benign tumors, it can be an important noninvasive method to make the tumor stop growing. Radiation therapy does have side effects as described earlier. Having a treatment team that will help make decisions about radiation is an important part of informed care in brain tumor therapy.

13

—◼—

Chemotherapy

I didn't know what chemotherapy was. I never knew how it would feel. I had no clue. I found out the hard way and the best way. It sure worked.

To be honest, it really wasn't all that difficult. I was preparing myself for the worst. They always gave me anti-nausea medication. I wasn't in the hospital overnight. I'm very glad I did it, and I always consider it a round, like a boxing match. If the tumor ever comes back, I'll do it again. I'm ready and that will be round two.

—Arthur (A.J.) Kirwan, diagnosed with a Grade III astrocytoma eleven years ago

For many people, the word *chemotherapy* is linked to visions of bald patients who are terribly sick from medications that essentially poison the whole body. Today there are major improvements in chemotherapy such that most regimens are very well tolerated.

We recommend chemotherapy in addition to radiation for malignant gliomas (including glioblastoma multiforme) and it is usually the mainstay of treatment for recurrent gliomas.

Should I Have Chemotherapy?

The decision about whether to try chemotherapy depends on each individual's situation. We weigh the risks and benefits of this treatment carefully for each person. We can give a single chemotherapy drug or a combination of drugs to treat brain tumors. Chemotherapy may also be given alone or in combination with surgery or radiation therapy.

Note: Drs. Patrick Wen and Jan Drappatz of Dana-Farber/ Brigham and Women's Cancer Center were of great help in the writing of this chapter and the next.

Depending on the type of chemotherapy and your treatment plan, you will take these drugs at home, in an outpatient clinic, or in the hospital. These are all considerations that may affect whether or not you want to pursue chemotherapy as a treatment option.

The decision to undergo chemotherapy isn't a simple one. In addition to the well-known, standard treatments, new drugs are being developed and new clinical trials for drugs are opening up all the time. The decision about which type of drug regimen to pursue can be daunting. Lisa Doherty, an oncology nurse practitioner in our brain tumor group, says, "Our patients often ask, 'If you were in my shoes, what would you do?' That's a difficult question to answer. In some ways, we are biased: we know our studies, but not necessarily the studies that other medical centers are doing. It's hard to place ourselves in our patients' shoes because everyone has different priorities. I emphasize quality of life as well as quantity."

When considering your chemotherapy options, ask about the drug's main side effects. Although you will find a long list of cautions on the drug's packaging, in consent forms for treatment, and in the chief reference book on medications for health care providers—*The Physician's Desk Reference*—no one experiences every side effect on the list. Some side effects will apply to most people who take the drug; others occur just once in every 100 patients. Ask your nurse or doctor which side effects she or he sees most commonly.

Also consider which clinical trials you have access to, and make an informed decision, but don't waste too much time wading through an overwhelming amount of information. Trust that you've chosen the right team of physicians to help guide you. You will find more information about how clinical trials work in chapter 14.

Terms You May Hear

Adjuvant chemotherapy: Given in addition to radiation therapy or surgery.

Alkaloid: An organic substance that contains nitrogen; alkaloid medications are often derived from seed plants.

Anti-angiogenic chemotherapy: Works by cutting off the tumor's ability to grow by forming new blood vessels.

Apoptosis (programmed cell death): A normal sequence of steps at a molecular level that leads to the death of an extra or abnormal cell. In tumor cells, this series of steps may be blocked; this blockage enables bad cells to thrive and replicate themselves.

Blood-brain barrier: Normally the endothelial cells that line the brain's blood vessels protect the brain from noxious body substances by preventing them from passing from the bloodstream to the brain. Chemotherapy drugs must pass through this barrier in order to reach brain tumors.

Cytostatic: Something that stops the reproduction of tumor cells and the growth of tumors but does not kill the cells.

Cytotoxic: Something that kills cells.

Drug resistant: Cancer cells that do not respond to chemotherapy.

High-dose chemotherapy: Treatment that is intense enough to destroy both cancer cells and bone marrow. This chemotherapy is often followed by a bone marrow "rescue" or stem-cell transplant to replenish the cells of the bone marrow with the person's own cryopreserved (frozen) bone marrow cells.

Low-dose (metronomic) chemotherapy: Frequent doses of small amounts of chemotherapy. Low-dose chemotherapy is often combined with other treatments like radiation therapy.

Per os (PO): By mouth.

Receptor-mediated permeabilizers: Substances that allow drugs to pass through openings in the blood-brain barrier.

How Chemotherapy Works

Chemotherapy drugs directly attack brain tumor cells and prevent them from dividing and spreading. If the cells cannot divide, a tumor cannot grow. For this reason, we use chemotherapy to treat malignant brain tumors exclusively.

In this chapter, I will describe the types of chemotherapy that the Food and Drug Administration (FDA) has approved to treat various forms of brain tumors. You will first see the standard (generic) name for the drug, followed by its trade name. I also will describe how chemotherapy is administered, how long the treatment cycles last, and what kinds of side effects and recuperation period you can expect. In chapter 14, you will find more information about new (novel) chemotherapy drugs under development and other chemotherapy drugs that have been approved by the FDA for the treatment of other types of tumors. We sometimes use these drugs on an "off-label" basis to fight brain tumors as well; that is, we use them for tumors that the FDA has not specifically said they are approved for.

How Chemotherapy Is Administered

Usually a neuro-oncologist (a specialist in cancers of the nervous system or a cancer specialist who treats brain tumors with medications) or a general oncologist (a medical doctor who specializes in the treatment of cancer of all types) administers chemotherapy. As I mentioned earlier, your doctor may recommend a single drug or a combination of chemotherapy drugs to fight your tumor.

The frequency and length of the treatments will also vary depending on the type of tumor and how it is responding to treatment. People take "cycles" of chemotherapy: they take the drug for one or for a few days and then take a break so that their healthy tissues can recover by creating new cells. This treatment-rest cycle is often repeated over many months.

You may take chemotherapy through a vein, by mouth, through an artery, directly into the cerebrospinal fluid, or (after surgery) directly into the part of your brain where the tumor was removed:

Injection into a vein (intravenously). Intravenous (IV) chemotherapy is the most common form of chemotherapy delivery. It is usually given in an outpatient setting—you won't need to be admitted to the hospital for this treatment.

By mouth (orally). Some chemotherapy drugs are given in pill or capsule form.

Injection into an artery (intra-arterially). Injection of chemotherapy drugs into an artery is associated with greater toxicity to the brain and eye than IV injection. Perhaps for that reason, it has fallen out of favor.

Injection into the cerebrospinal fluid (intrathecally, intraventricularly). Rarely, an oncologist will ask to have chemotherapy delivered directly into the ventricular system of the brain (as you will recall from chapter 1, this is a system of "great lakes" that contain cerebrospinal fluid). For this type of injection, a small bubble or reservoir is placed under your scalp; it creates a bump from which cerebrospinal fluid can be withdrawn. Chemotherapy drugs also can be injected into this reservoir; from there they travel to the ventricle.

Administration into the tumor site or directly into the tumor (interstitial or intratumoral chemotherapy). After an operation to remove a brain tumor, neurosurgeons sometimes implant a chemotherapy-soaked wafer directly into the brain. The wafer dissolves gradually and doesn't have to be removed. The wafer most commonly used is called Gliadel, which contains the chemotherapeutic agent BCNU.

This technique is beneficial because the chemotherapy drug can be delivered without concern about its ability to cross the blood-brain barrier. Also, because the concentrated drug is placed right into the tumor bed, it is less toxic to other areas of the brain. However, this form of chemotherapy may make a patient ineligible for further chemotherapy trials. Speak with your oncologist and surgeon prior to surgery if you are interested in pursuing clinical trials after surgery.

Researchers are also exploring ways to insert other chemotherapy agents directly into brain tumors. For more information about this novel form of therapy, see chapter 14. The benefits of this therapy are that the treatment goes straight to the tumor.

Chemotherapy for Brain Tumors in Children

As I will explain in greater detail in chapter 17, chemotherapy is the preferable treatment for brain tumors in infants and children under age three because radiation can be harmful to the developing brain.

Five chemotherapy drugs that are given to children are:

1. *vincristine (Oncovin),* a natural alkaloid-derived agent that kills dividing cells. This drug, which is given intravenously, does not affect blood cell counts as dramatically as many other chemotherapy drugs.
2. *cisplatin (Platinol),* a form of platinum that can destroy tumor cells and prevent tumor growth. It is given intravenously and can cause nausea, tingling, or numbness in the hands or feet (peripheral neuropathy), and, rarely, damage to the kidneys.

3. **procarbazine (Matulane)** works by damaging the DNA of tumor cells and is given intravenously, usually once a month. It can make blood counts fall.

4. **methotrexate (Abitrexate, Folex, Mexate, Rheumatrex)** affects cell metabolism and is given intravenously. It can have significant adverse effects on the white matter of the brain; this can cause learning difficulties.

5. **temozolomide (Methazolastone, Temodar)** is an alkylating agent first used in adults with brain tumors and now increasingly used in children. It can be given orally a few days each month for years.

Chemotherapy for Brain Tumors in Adults

A number of agents are used for brain tumors in adults. Some of these are used alone and others are used in combination with other drugs.

Single-Agent Chemotherapy

- **temozolomide (Methazolastone, Temodar)** is an alkylating agent that received an accelerated approval by the FDA in 1999 because of its good results in patients with malignant primary brain tumors. It crosses the blood-brain barrier and is 100 percent bioavailable—that is, it is well absorbed into the rest of the body through the gastrointestinal tract.

  For: This drug is showing promise for the long-term management of gliomas; it may be useful in medulloblastomas and metastatic tumors.

  Administered: In one to six oral capsules a few days (often five days) per month for a year or more. Treatment-rest cycles can last for several months or years.

  Considerations: Although temozolomide is often well tolerated, it can cause fatigue, nausea, vomiting, and constipation. Your blood counts will need to be monitored carefully while you are taking this drug.

- **carmustine (BCNU, Becenum, BiCNU, Carmubris)**, a nitrosourea agent (a type of anti-tumor drug), can cross the blood-brain barrier, disrupt the DNA of tumor cells, and stop these cells from proliferating.

For: Anaplastic gliomas and glioblastomas.

Administered: Intravenously on an outpatient basis for 90 minutes; the cycle repeats every six weeks.

Considerations: Some people feel a burning sensation when carmustine is going into a vein. Nausea, vomiting, fatigue, constipation, and diarrhea are also common. Your blood counts will need to be monitored carefully while you are taking this drug.

- **lomustine (CCNU, CeeNU),** is a nitrosourea (an anti-tumor drug) like BCNU that can cross the blood-brain barrier and stop cancer cells from spreading by inhibiting their DNA and RNA synthesis. It can be given orally.

  For: Anaplastic gliomas and glioblastoma.

  Administered: Orally.

  Considerations: This drug has the same side effects as BCNU.

- **procarbazine (Matulane),** rarely used alone, is most often taken in combination with CCNU and vincristine in a chemotherapy regimen called PCV.

  For: Malignant gliomas.

  Administered: Orally.

  Considerations: PCV was the first drug combination shown to have efficacy in anaplastic oligodendrogliomas with a chromosomal loss in chromosome 1 and 19 (a 1p19q deletion).

- **polifeprosan 20 with carmustine (BCNU) implant (Gliadel wafer)**

  For: Malignant gliomas.

  Administered: In a biodegradable wafer that is implanted directly in the brain after surgery to remove a brain tumor. This wafer contains the chemotherapy drug carmustine (BCNU).

  Considerations: BCNU, when given in this form, does not affect blood counts as dramatically as it can when administered intravenously.

- **methotrexate (Trexall)**

  For: Lymphomas and medulloblastomas.

  Administered: Orally, intravenously, intra-arterially, or intrathecally.

  Considerations: As in children, methotrexate in adults can cause a drop in white blood cell counts and changes in brain white matter.

- **cis-retinoic acid (Accutane) or trans-retinoic acid**

  For: Anaplastic astrocytomas.

Administered: By mouth.

Considerations: This agent enhances programmed cell death (apoptosis) and has had some results in fighting anaplastic gliomas.

Chemotherapy with More than One Drug (Combination Chemotherapy)

- **procarbazine + lomustine (CCNU) + vincristine = PCV,** a common, bioavailable chemotherapy regimen.

  For: Both low-grade and malignant gliomas, any anaplastic brain tumors.

  Administered: Procarbazine and CCNU are oral medications; vincristine is given intravenously. The combination is usually given over a 28-day cycle: for instance, oral CCNU and intravenous anti-nausea medication on day 1; procarbazine at home for two weeks starting on day 8; and vincristine on days 8 and 29.

  Considerations: PCV can lower your blood counts. You may also experience fatigue, nerve discomfort (neuropathy), constipation, ringing in your ears, and jaw pain. Talk with your health care team about your diet while you are taking procarbazine.

- **ifosfamide (Cyfos, Ifex, Ifosfamidum) with cisplatin** works by preventing DNA replication in tumor cells. This regimen can be toxic to the kidneys and bladder, so a drug called mesna (Mesnex) is often given with this combination chemotherapy to protect the renal system.

  For: Medulloblastomas.

  Administered: Ifosfamide and cisplatin are given intravenously. Mesna may be taken by mouth or intravenously.

  Considerations: This therapy can cause kidney damage.

- **carboplatin, cis-retinoic acid (Accutane)** works by suppressing growth.

  For: Malignant gliomas.

  Administered: Carboplatin is given intravenously once a month; cis-retinoic acid is given in pill form every day.

  Considerations: This therapy combines an agent that promotes cell death (apoptosis) with an agent that stops cell division.

- **temozolomide (Temodar) with other drugs.** In an attempt to combine the benefits of temozolomide with other nontoxic agents, several combinations have been suggested, including:

- *temozolomide plus cis-retinoic acid (Accutane)*
- *temozolomide plus irinotecan (CPT-11)*

In chapter 14, I will tell you about combinations of some of these chemotherapy drugs (such as temozolomide) with many other drugs that have been approved by the FDA to treat conditions other than brain tumors. When these agents are used to treat brain tumors, we say that they are being used "off-label."

Side Effects of Chemotherapy

Traditional chemotherapy affects the division of all rapidly dividing cells in the body, including healthy cells that tend to replicate quickly, such as those in the bone marrow (where red and white blood cells and platelets are produced), hair, and the lining of the gastrointestinal tract. That is why this form of treatment can cause blood cell counts to plummet, hair to fall out, and patients to experience nausea, vomiting, and diarrhea. No one wants to feel sick, and doctors are constantly looking into new ways to stimulate your appetite, counteract your fatigue, and ease your discomfort while you go through this form of treatment.

Chemotherapy can also affect the cells in your heart, lungs, renal system (your kidneys and bladder), and nervous system. But the good news is that we now have many medications that are very effective in countering these side effects. Some people also try complementary therapies such as acupuncture and meditation (see chapter 18) to manage discomfort at this time. It may help to think of chemotherapy as a weapon against the brain tumor that you are fighting. One of my patients even dressed up as a gladiator when she came to the hospital for infusions of chemotherapy.

Nausea and Vomiting

Ask your health care team about anti-nausea medication that you can take even before your chemotherapy begins. Effective drugs like odansetron (Zofran) and granisetron (Kytril) can head off this side effect. Sedative agents like lorazepam (Ativan) and diphenhydramine (Benadryl) also have a quieting effect on the nerves that cause nausea.

Diarrhea

Some people take antidiarrheal medications like loperamide (Imodium) or diphenoxylate hydrochloride and atropine (Lomotil) before they begin chemotherapy. However, you may not be able to take this kind of medication if you already have a gastrointestinal infection. Talk with your health care team.

Constipation

Some chemotherapy drugs can have the opposite effect—they can make you constipated. Laxatives and stool softeners can help. Be sure to drink lots of liquids.

Fatigue

Fatigue may be caused by both the cellular fight between the chemotherapy drug and the tumor and a low red blood cell count (anemia) due to chemotherapy's damage to the cells of the bone marrow. Your body will require extra energy to repair chemotherapy's damage to its tissues. Eating less because of nausea and other gastrointestinal effects may also make you tired.

Give yourself permission to take naps frequently. Napping does not mean that you are giving in to the tumor—it means that you are allowing your body to regroup to continue fighting it.

You may also find that a mild to moderate amount of exercise (10 minutes three times a day; 15 minutes twice a day; or 30 minutes once a day) three to four times a week can also improve your energy level.

If your fatigue persists, your health care team may prescribe:

- *modafinil (Provigil).* This stimulant can improve your energy level; however, it may reduce the effectiveness of other medications you are taking (such as anticonvulsants, antibiotics, and sometimes chemotherapy drugs). It also causes headache and sleeplessness in some people.
- *methylphenidate (Ritalin),* can also wake you up and make you feel better. Talk with your doctor about every other drug you are taking before you begin to take Ritalin, especially if you are taking the chemotherapy drug procarbazine (Matulane) or temozolomide (Temodar). People with glaucoma, Tourette's syndrome, some

allergies, and/or anxiety should not take this drug. Uncommon side effects resemble those you may experience when you drink too much coffee: a racing heartbeat, insomnia, and agitation.

- **methylphenidate HCl (Concerta)** and amphetamine mixed salts (**Adderall**) also increase alertness.

Low Blood Counts

Chemotherapy can affect both your white cell and red cell counts, so your health care team will monitor your blood counts often while you are taking chemotherapy drugs. If your red blood cell count is low, you may need a blood transfusion. If your white blood cell count is low, your health care provider may prescribe pegfilgrastim (Neulasta or Neupogen) to increase this count.

Fever

Just as the chemotherapy drug is destroying the cells in your brain tumor, it may be disrupting the growth of cells in your bone marrow, where blood cells, including white blood cells (neutrophils, lymphocytes, and monocytes) are produced. If your white blood cell count is low (neutropenia), you may be at risk for a throat, urinary tract, or other type of infection.

Avoid crowded, closed-in places like schools and movie theaters while your risk of infection is increased. Wash your hands often and be careful about using an antiseptic over superficial scrapes or cuts. Let someone else change the baby's diaper or pick up after the dog.

If you feel unwell, check your temperature. You may have a low-grade fever simply because your metabolism is "kicked up" in its fight against the tumor cells. However, if your fever is 100.5 or higher, call your nurse or doctor, especially if you just don't feel right and you can't attribute your fatigue to something else (like insufficient sleep).

Hair Loss

Many people who take chemotherapy drugs for a brain tumor do not lose their hair. Those who do may find that their hair becomes thinner before it gradually falls out or comes out in clumps. Just as with radiation treatment, hair loss associated with chemotherapy may not happen immediately. Then eyelashes, pubic hair, and hair elsewhere on the body may stop growing for a while. When it returns, it may be thicker or a slightly different color than it was before. You may need to protect yourself from the sun for many months after your chemotherapy ends.

A lot of people wear scarves and hats to cover their heads when their hair is thin. If you choose to wear a hair prosthesis or wig, see a wigmaker before you begin treatment. Many insurance plans will cover up to $500 of the cost. Today there are high-quality wigs that are so natural that most people won't notice them.

Sore Mouth

Chemotherapy sometimes causes bleeding and stomatitis, inflammation of the mucous membranes inside the mouth. Before you begin chemotherapy treatment, you may wish to see your dentist for a checkup and get advice about mouth care during this time.

We recommend that patients use a soft toothbrush or even a facecloth to clean their teeth if their gums are sensitive. You may use a saltwater rinse as well, but don't use a mouthwash that contains alcohol—it may dry your mouth.

If you develop uncomfortable sores in your mouth, prescription medications such as nystatin can help. You may also want to try a prescription mouthwash called "Miracle mouthwash," a one-to-one solution of (Maalox), lidocaine, and diphenhydramine (Benadryl).

Bleeding

A low blood platelet count (thrombocytopenia) from chemotherapy can lead to unexpected bleeding or bruising. Tell your health-care team if you notice blood in your urine or bowel movements. If your platelet count is too low, you may need to have a transfusion to replace them.

Other Things to Consider

Alcohol and other drugs can interfere with chemotherapy, so avoid alcohol at this time and be sure to tell your health-care team about every type of medicine you may be taking, even if it's an over-the-counter vitamin or supplement. Some people are so used to taking medicines for high blood pressure or hormone replacement therapy that they don't think of them as being drugs.

Chemotherapy can also affect a person's fertility, so talk with your health care team about freezing your eggs or sperm for the future if you are planning to have children.

New Therapies

Researchers are actively seeking ways to overcome the resistance of some tumors to chemotherapy. For instance, if we can disable one of their DNA repair genes such as MGMT, gliomas may be more responsive to alkylating agents like Temodar. Scientists are also investigating combinations of chemotherapy drugs with angiogenesis inhibitors (that is, drugs that inhibit the ability of tumors to feed themselves by creating new blood vessels) like thalidomide (see chapter 14).

Chemotherapy drugs such as Temodar may also be combined with targeted molecular drugs such as gefitinib (Iressa), erlotinib (Tarceva), and lenalidomide (Revlimid).

Chemotherapy can be an important treatment for some brain tumors and some new agents do not have the infamous severe side effects of those used in the past. In the next chapter, I will tell you about new drug therapies as well as some of the drugs that are often paired with chemotherapy drugs in the treatment of brain tumors.

14

—■—

Newer Therapies

As we have seen, there are several established, proven methods of treating brain tumors. It's important to realize that many of those treatments didn't exist ten years ago—and doctors continue to pioneer advances in treatment, uncovering new research discoveries every day. This suggests that we are moving closer and closer to our ultimate goal: developing a cure for brain tumors.

Several new treatments on the horizon for brain tumors show increasing effectiveness. These include new general chemotherapy drugs; anti-angiogenic therapy (therapy directed at cutting off the blood supply to tumors); anti-growth factor therapy; immunotherapy; targeted molecular therapies; and new local therapies.

As you consider your treatment options, ask your doctor about experimental therapies. You might be able to participate in a clinical trial for a drug or treatment method that is under development. Alternatively, drug companies may offer so-called *novel* or *off-label drugs* at or reduced cost if you cannot afford them otherwise (see www.helpingpatients.org). The FDA has not approved these drugs, so they may not be covered by your insurance. Most of these agents are being used for malignant gliomas.

Novel Approaches to Malignant Gliomas

Traditional chemotherapeutic agents selectively kill cells that are dividing. Newer agents may kill dividing cells, stop new blood vessel formation, enhance the body's immune response, cause differentiation of tumor cells, or target specific growth factors. This section lists some of these drugs—it is not meant to be a comprehensive list but gives some sense of the range of possible agents presently available. Some new drugs have had good success in other cancers and are just now being considered for brain tumors.

Drugs That Stop Cell Division

- *carboplatin (Paraplat, Paraplatin),* like its parent compound, cisplatin, kills dividing tumor cells. It is less toxic and more stable than cisplatin. Carboplatin, used for malignant gliomas, is given intravenously once a month. In a few patients it may cause shortness of breath and chest pain within the first fifteen minutes of infusion. If this happens, carboplatin therapy should be discontinued. This drug can also cause nausea and vomiting. A close relative of this drug, *oxaliplatin* (*Eloxatin*), is also being used for glioblastoma treatment.
- *irinotecan (Camptosar, CPT-11)* is derived from camptothecin, an alkaloid substance that comes from the Asian tree *Camptotheca acuminata* and is toxic to cells. It has recently been combined with temozolomide (Temodar) for treatment of glioblastomas intravenously weekly for three weeks. This combination therapy can cause mild to severe diarrhea, nausea, vomiting, blood clots, fatigue, and thinning of hair.
- *tamoxifen (Nolvadex),* a drug used to fight breast cancer, can inhibit the division of brain tumor cells by interfering with an enzyme called protein kinase C. It is used to fight glioblastomas and anaplastic astrocytomas and is administered by mouth. Tamoxifen can cause nausea, weight gain, and blood clots.
- *pyrazoloacridine (PZA, 366140),* a drug that kills dividing cells, is being studied as an agent to fight glioblastoma multiforme and a childhood cancer called neuroblastoma.

- *flavopiridol* is being used for germ-cell tumors.
- *karenitecin (BNP1350, 710270),* like irinotecan, is derived from camptothecin, which is toxic to dividing cancer cells.
- *arsenic trioxide* is an agent that enhances programmed cell death.
- *BMS-247550* is a microtubule stabilizer that diminishes cell division; it keeps the cell structure stable so there is less likelihood that the cells will divide.

The promise of these drugs is that they can provide specific blockades to brain tumor growth. They may act as a "magic bullet" that will kill only tumor cells and leave normal brain cells alone.

Anti-Angiogenic Therapy

Recently, doctors have been researching an especially promising biological therapy for brain tumors involving angiogenesis inhibitors, drugs that disrupt the growth of blood vessels that feed tumors. *Angiogenesis* refers to the formation of new blood vessels by brain tumors. *Anti-angiogenic therapy* cuts off the tumor's supply of blood, oxygen, and vital nutrients and in doing so prevents its growth. This type of therapy is being investigated for malignant gliomas, which thrive on a rich blood supply and can be very aggressive. These drugs include:

- *thalidomide (Synovir, Thalomid).* You may remember this drug because it was associated with birth defects when it was used as a sleeping medicine in the late 1950s. Some babies were born without limbs because of the interruption in their blood supply after their mothers had taken thalidomide. Today we know that this agent can also interfere with the blood supply that feeds tumors. For management of brain tumors, thalidomide may be helpful when it is combined with other drugs (such as BCNU, a chemotherapy drug) and/or radiation therapy. Side effects of thalidomide include constipation and fatigue.
- *lenalidomide (Revlimid, CC5013).* Lenalidomide does not have the sedating effects of thalidomide, but it shares the same risk of causing birth defects.
- *cyclooxygenase-2 (COX-2) inhibitors (Celebrex, SC-58635,*

719627). COX-2 inhibition may stimulate programmed cell death (apoptosis), thereby reducing the tumor's angiogenesis and metastasis. These nonsteroidal anti-inflammatory drugs may be combined with temozolomide (Temodar).

- *platelet factor 4 (PF4).* This commercially available anti-angiogenic agent is derived from platelets and is very expensive because of its manufacturing process.
- *pegylated interferon alfa (PEG-IFNa).* This combination of interferon alpha (IFNa) and polyethylene glycol (PEG) is more effective than either of these compounds alone.
- *SU5416.* Vascular endothelial growth factor (VEGF) is one of the most potent factors a tumor uses to draw blood vessels into it. SU5416 is a targeted therapeutic agent that blocks the receptor for VEGF and other growth factors. This means that a tumor cannot effectively attract blood vessels into it, and therefore dies.
- *AZD2171.* By inhibiting VEGF receptors, this agent blocks both angiogenesis and the growth of tumor cells.
- *endostatin.* A nonspecific anti-angiogenesis agent that is difficult to manufacture but appears to have a very important ability to block angiogenesis.
- *bevacizumab (Avastin).* A so-called recombinant humanized monoclonal antibody that prevents the growth of tumor blood vessels by blocking VEGF, one of the factors that brain tumors use to attract new blood vessels.

The possibility that we can use anti-angiogenesis agents to starve a tumor is an exciting idea that is just now being worked on in clinical trials.

Differentiating Agents

Another way to inhibit tumor growth is to change the cells themselves from immature cells that divide to mature cells that do not divide. The process by which a tumor cell diverges from the life cycle of a normal cell and becomes malignant is called *dedifferentiation.* Drugs that interrupt this process and lead to a stable, differentiated cell include:

- *bryostatin 1 (B705008K112, 339555),* a substance that is derived from aquatic organisms called bryozoan Bugula neritina, stops the dedifferentiation and proliferation of tumor cells by interfering with the cell-signaling enzyme protein kinase C. Bryostatin may work well with other chemotherapy drugs.
- *retinoic acid (13-cis-retinoic acid) (Accutane),* an oral medication for the treatment of acne, can also block the endothelial growth factor receptor (EGFR), which is used by many tumors to grow. Side effects of this drug include nausea and headache. Retinoic acid is also associated with a risk of birth defects.

Immunotherapy

Immunotherapy can improve the immune system's ability to locate and destroy tumor cells. As our understanding of the underlying mechanisms controlling immune reactions within the brain grows, we may develop more effective therapies against brain tumors in the future. Immunotherapeutic agents include interferons (IF), natural proteins that are toxic to cancerous cells, and specific antibodies. Interferons stimulate the production of B cells, which attack tumors. Alpha, beta, and gamma are the three families of interferon. Promising new agents include:

- *recombinant interferon beta, interferon beta 1-a, and interferon beta 1-b (Betaseron, Rebif)* are oral agents that may be used to fight anaplastic astrocytomas and glioblastomas.
- *interleukins (IL)* stimulate the production of immune cells that can kill cancer cells. They are numbered IL-1 through IL-15. Several of them have potential in the treatment of tumors.
- *tumor vaccines* are made by removing cells from the tumor, enhancing their ability to kill tumor cells, and putting them back directly into the tumor. Dendritic cells are one example of this kind of immunotherapy; these cells are immune cells that can be trained to fight brain tumors specifically. Once these cells are modified, they will not grow when they are reintroduced to the person's body; rather, they will help his or her immune system fight the tumor.
- *IL-13 PE38QQR (IL-13-pseudomonas exotoxin)* can be attached to

immune cells to kill the tumor once the immune cells have identified the tumor. A national trial in the treatment of glioblastomas recently showed that this exotoxin could be administered through a catheter, into the tumor directly.

- **transferrin receptor and pseudomonas exotoxin (transMID, transferrin-CRM107, HN-66000),** a targeted synthetic protein toxin, is made of human transferrin (a protein that attaches itself to and is absorbed by tumor cells) and a diphtheria toxin (CRM107). The toxin enters the tumor cells and kills them. These types of drugs are called *ligand-targeted toxin conjugates.*
- **radionuclides such as I-131 TM-601 (scorpion venom clorotoxin)** are radiopharmaceuticals containing a synthetic version of chlorotoxin, a substance derived from scorpion venom; these agents bind to a receptor expressed on tumor cells, but not on normal cells.

For many years, there has been great interest in enhancing immune responses to malignant brain tumors. These new approaches renew that interest in an important way.

Terms You May Hear: Immunotherapy

Biologic response modifier (BRM): An agent (or a natural substance) that is used to stop the growth of a tumor by building up or replacing normal immune defenses. Interferons are naturally produced BRMs that interfere with cell division. Interleukins are also naturally occurring BRMs.

Biologic therapy: The use of biologic response modifiers (BRMs) to make the body less favorable to the growth of tumors.

Immunotoxin: These attach a toxic or radioactive antibody to a tumor cell. Once the antibody identifies the cell as abnormal, it will destroy it. Researchers are investigating ways to deliver immunotoxins directly into brain tumors (intratumoral therapy).

Lymphocytes: White blood cells that produce antibodies; they are an important part of the immune system.

Lymphokine-activated killer (LAK) cells: Lymphocytes that have been manipulated in the laboratory so that they attack tumor cells.

Gene Therapy

Gene therapy is the transfer of genetic material into a tumor cell to destroy the cell or to stop cell growth. Numerous types of genes are under investigation, including those that signal tumor cells to self-destruct; genes that make cells more mature (skipping stages of cell growth); genes that can strengthen the immune system's attack on the tumor; and genes that increase the cell's responsiveness to certain drugs.

Viruses are one method doctors use to insert foreign genetic material into cells—viruses attach to a cell and inject their material. By modifying a particular virus, tumor cells can be selectively damaged. The major challenge is making sure that the virus does not affect normal cells. Gene therapy viruses or "vectors" can be administered by way of a stereotactic injection directly into the tumor; this injection delivers the virus into very specific areas of the tumor. Gene therapies may use a gene that destroys both the virus and the tumor cell; this "suicide gene" contains a compound that, when exposed to a drug the patient takes, becomes toxic to the cells involved.

Recently our laboratory and others have investigated the use of stem cells as gene therapy agents. Unlike viruses, they will track down the tumor cells and can thereby act as "smart" gene therapy agents, killing themselves and the tumor cells when they are exposed to an external agent that causes them to self-destruct.

Terms You May Hear: Gene Therapy

Antisense therapies: Drugs that interfere with the protein messages created by malignant cells. This type of gene therapy is designed to block the growth of a tumor by "disconnecting" these protein messages.

Bystander effect: A phenomenon noted in gene therapy in which not only the targeted cell but also the cells around it may be destroyed by one viral infection.

Interference RNA: A new kind of treatment that can prevent RNA, which provides the blueprint for cell division, from acting effectively. It neutralizes the tumor cell's RNA and thereby stops growth.

Targeted Molecular Therapies

Researchers are exploring the possibility of blocking specific growth pathways that a tumor cell may use. Normal cells use different pathways than tumor cells, so these drugs block just the tumor cell pathways—sparing those of the normal cells.

The concept is quite simple: find out what growth factors the cell uses, then block them and watch the cell stop growing. Specific molecules are used to block cell growth (hence "molecular therapy"). This therapy is particularly attractive because it should not affect normal cells. Unlike chemotherapy drugs, which inhibit the growth of any dividing cells in the body, targeted molecular therapies zero in on just the tumor cells, so the healthy cells in the body aren't threatened.

Targeted molecular therapies such as Gleevec, Tarceva, Iressa, and Avastin, which were originally designed to attack the molecular abnormalities of other types of tumor cells (for instance, in the lung, colon, breast, and prostate) are now being given to some patients with brain tumors. In particular, glioblastoma multiforme shares some of the molecular abnormalities of other types of tumors in the body.

Normal cells produce proteins called *growth factors*. Brain tumors produce too many of these proteins. Small molecular inhibitors of tumor growth factors such as epidermal growth factor (EGF) and platelet-derived growth factor (PDGF) receptors are showing some promise in research studies. They are particularly effective when the molecular target (the growth factor) is driving the tumor's growth and when the drug can reach and inhibit the target at doses that drastically reduce the proportion of receptors fueling growth.

Researchers have found that these agents are more effective when used in combination with each other and with radiation and chemotherapy. Chemotherapy drugs such as temozolomide (Temodar) thus may be combined with targeted molecular drugs such as PTK 787, Iressa or Tarceva, SCH6618 or R115777, RAD001, and lenalidomide (Revlimid).

Epidermal Growth Factor Receptor (EGFR) Antagonists

Primary glioblastomas have cells with molecular abnormalities that change, amplify, and overexpress epidermal growth factor receptor

(EGFR; also called ErbB1 or HER1), the protein on the surface of some cells. When epidermal growth factor attaches itself to this protein, the cells divide. There are too many EGFRs on the surface of many kinds of tumor cells, so they have the ability to divide quickly. Researchers are investigating therapies that can target EGFR. Existing targeted therapies to inhibit the EGFR of malignant gliomas include:

- *gefitinib (Iressa, ZD1839).* May arrest the cell cycle and stop angiogenesis; side effects may include rash and nausea, vomiting, and diarrhea.
- *erlotinib (Tarceva, OSI-774,718781), erlotinib hydrochloride.* This drug is a similar to gefitinib.
- *lapatinib (GW-572016, GW2016).* Currently in clinical trials for its effectiveness against solid tumors. Common side effects of this drug are diarrhea and a rash.

Platelet-Derived Growth Factor (PDGF) Antagonists

The cells of low-grade astrocytomas tend to produce too much of the protein called platelet-derived growth factor (PDGF) and its receptors (PDGFR). Targeted therapies to inhibit the PDGF of malignant gliomas include:

- *Imatinib mesylate (STI 571, Gleevec).* Gleevec, the first targeted molecular therapy, was developed in 2001 for patients who were suffering from chronic myelogenous leukemia (CML) and produced astonishing results. It is now being given to patients with malignant gliomas.

Vascular Endothelial Growth Factor Receptor (VEGF) Inhibitors

Drugs that inhibit the production of another protein, called VEGF, may control both the angiogenesis and swelling around malignant gliomas:

- *bevacizumab (Avastin).* A drug that blocks VEGF receptors and therefore blood vessel formation.
- *PTK787 (ZK222584).* A targeted molecule against several growth factors.

Mammalian Target of Rapamycin (mTOR) Inhibitors

Drugs that inhibit the mammalian target of rapamycin (mTOR) enzyme (a protein essential for cell survival and tumor growth) disrupt the progression of the cell cycle. Some mTOR inhibitors that are currently under investigation include:

- *temsirolimus (CCI-779, 683864)*
- *everolimus (Certican, RAD001)*
- *sirolimus (rapamycin, Rapamune, 226080),* derived from the bacterium *Streptomyces hygroscopicus,* also has immunosuppressant properties.

Laser Photoactivation/Photodynamic Radiation Therapy (PRT or PDT)

During laser photoactivation, a drug called a hematoporphyrin derivative is injected through a vein and is taken up by the tumor cells. When these cells are subsequently exposed to light during laser surgery, the drug is activated, killing the cells. However, the range of penetration is not very great for this therapy and it therefore is best for treating the region around a tumor. Difficulties include identifying a truly selective dye that will only be absorbed by cancer cells and delivering the laser energy effectively over the entire tumor.

Intratumoral Therapies

An important new concept in brain tumor therapy is to insert some of the new biological therapies directly into the tumor. Many drugs in the blood cannot get into the brain because it is a protected environment, so this insertion of intratumoral agents allows much less of a drug to be used and may increase effective therapy. Our laboratory and others have evaluated anti-angiogenic agents and anti-invasiveness agents given by direct infusion into the tumor or placed in polymers that are left in the tumor bed after surgery. Some of the compounds that are being tested against malignant gliomas are:

- *131-I monoclonal antibody 3F8 against GD2,* which attempts to block growth.
- *131-I monoclonal antibody 81C6 anti-Tenascin,* which attempts to block invasion.
- *mafosfamid,* used with chemotherapy and radiation.
- *topotecan (Hycamtin),* a Topoisomerase I inhibitor.
- *infusion of TP-38,* pseudomonas exotoxin linked to TGF-a targeting EGFR. This molecule is used locally to inhibit tumor growth within the tumor.
- *convection-enhanced delivery of IL 13-PE38QQR,* pseudomonas exotoxin linked to IL 13.
- *busulfan (Busulfex, Mitosan, Myleran),* for medulloblastomas and supratentorial primitive neuroectodermal tumors.

Clinical Trials for New Brain Tumor Therapies

Clinical trials study the effectiveness of new drugs and procedures for the treatment of brain tumors. The goal, of course, is to find treatments that will stop the growth of tumors or shrink them. Researchers in clinical trials are also concerned with finding the appropriate dosages of new drugs and identifying possible side effects as well as the effect of the treatment on the patient's quality of life.

It is sometimes difficult to know which clinical trials are worth entering. The National Institutes of Health (NIH) endorses a consortia of hospitals/doctors for specific treatments. Many clinical trials for the treatment of brain tumors are carried out through consortium arrangements. These groups of hospitals join together to create combined trials of various agents and approaches. In the United States, there are two adult chemotherapy consortia—the North American Brain Tumor Consortium (NABTC) and New Approaches to Brain Tumor Therapy (NABTT). In addition to these, the Radiation Therapy Oncology Group (RTOG) examines the role of radiation therapy in treating tumors. In Europe, there is the EORTC, the European Organization for Research and Treatment of Cancer. For the study of treatments for brain tumors in children, there are the Pediatric Brain Tumor Consortium (PBTC) and the Children's Oncology Group (COG).

For treatment of recurrent or difficult to treat brain tumors, I recommend finding a brain tumor group at an institution near you that is a member of the NIH's consortia or another consortia. Another choice is to find an institution that has a comprehensive NIH-funded cancer center and work with its brain tumor center. Web sites that will be helpful in this type of research are listed in the Resources section at the end of this book.

As you consider entering a clinical trial, it is important to remember that you may not benefit from the drug or procedure under test. Depending on the phase of the trial, which I will describe below, it may take a long time before a drug becomes FDA approved.

As you are exploring your eligibility for a clinical trial, ask your doctor:

- Am I taking or have I taken any drugs that would prevent me from enrolling in this trial?
- Have I had or am I currently undergoing a form of therapy that would prevent me from enrolling in this trial?
- Will I have to pay for it or will insurance or a drug company cover the cost? Any therapy that is considered to be routine care is generally covered by insurance. Experimental drugs and procedures may not be covered. However, some parts of the clinical trial process (like certain tests before hospital admission testing) usually are covered. Drug companies and device manufacturers sometimes cover the cost of parking and in some trials provide a small stipend. Talk with your hospital's billing department to find out more about coverage for the trial you are considering.
- How long will this surgical or non-surgical procedure take? Will I be in pain? What are the known side effects of the drug?

Before you can participate in a clinical trial, you will need to read and sign a consent form. This form, though very detailed, is usually written in plain language. Be sure to ask questions about anything in the consent form that is not clear to you.

While you are part of a clinical trial, you may be considered a "subject"—not a "patient." When you go off the trial, you will again become a patient. This does not mean you will not be cared for during the clinical trial. You remain a person who is extremely important to the investigators.

To find out more about promising therapies and how to explore appropriate clinical trials to treat a brain tumor, look at www.ClinicalTrials.gov. You can also access Physician Data Query (PDQ), the database of ongoing clinical trials that are sponsored by the National Cancer Institute and other institutions: www.cancer.gov/cancer_information; or call 800-422-6237.

Terms You May Hear: Clinical Trials

Single-blind study: Patients do not know which arm of the clinical trial they are in; that is, whether they are receiving the standard therapy or the new drug. Their physicians have this information.

Double-blind study: Neither the patient nor his or her doctor knows whether the patient is receiving standard therapy or the new drug under study in a clinical trial.

Non-randomized study: In this type of clinical trial, all patients receive the same treatment.

Randomized study or randomized clinical trial (RCT): A clinical trial in which patients are assigned randomly to either a standard treatment "arm" or a treatment arm that includes the new drug under study. This is the best way to evaluate the effect of a new therapy.

Placebo study: A clinical trial that includes a placebo, an inactive, harmless substance, as part of its design. Most brain tumor clinical trials do not include a placebo arm, but instead compare the new drug with standard therapies.

Protocol: The plan for a clinical trial. The protocol details the number of patients who will participate, the tests they will undergo, and the treatment regimen.

Informed consent: A document that explains the risks and benefits of an experimental therapy. All patients who participate in federally regulated studies must sign this form to show that they have read and understand these risks and benefits.

Institutional Review Board (IRB): A committee of individuals who must approve the safety and design of clinical trial protocols that are conducted at their institution. This committee is usually composed of physicians, scientists, administrative people, and regular laypeople who offer their time for this important effort.

Intramural (from the Latin *intra*-"inside" and *mur*-"wall") *research.* Researchers whose laboratories are physically situated in the National Cancer Institute of the National Institutes of Health perform intramural research. *Extramural* research is conducted by researchers outside of the NCI at hospitals, universities, and laboratories.

Investigational new drug (IND): A drug that the Food and Drug Administration (FDA) has only approved for use in clinical trials.

New drug application (NDA): A drug company that wants FDA approval to sell a drug must first file an NDA.

Phase 1 Trials: Conducted to find out whether a drug is toxic. They are not meant to find out whether the drug is effective or not.

Phase 2 Trials: Establish the maximum tolerated dose (MTD) of a new drug. Usually 25 or fewer patients take the experimental treatment as part of the study's research into dosing and side effects.

Phase 3 Trials: Try to show that a treatment is effective and usually compare one drug against the standard treatment to show which works best.

Pilot study: A drug is given to a few patients to test for safety and efficacy before it is given to more patients.

Principal investigator (PI): The person responsible for the conduct of a study.

Research in Brain Tumors

In general, medical research can be divided into basic research (for example, a study of fundamental mechanisms of cell growth and division); clinical research (for example, a study of the effects of a particular drug on patients with brain tumors); and translational research (research that tries to move between basic science and clinical work). Translational research is particularly important for brain tumors, because it tries to apply ideas in basic science to actual treatment.

A decade ago, few laboratories were doing research in brain tumors. This has changed, thanks in large part to advocacy groups such as the

Brain Tumor Society, the American Brain Tumor Association, the Florida Brain Tumor Society, the Pediatric Brain Tumor Foundation, and collaborative efforts of all brain tumor support groups. Foundations like the Sontag Foundation, the McDonnell Foundation, the Goldhirsh Foundation, and ABC² (Accelerated Brain Cancer Care) also have a special brain tumor emphasis. These invaluable groups have heightened the awareness of brain tumors, have provided start-up grant funding, and have advocated at the NIH and elsewhere for greater funding for research into the treatment of these tumors.

An example of a translational brain tumor research laboratory is the Black Laboratory at Brigham and Women's Hospital in Boston, a laboratory I have directed since 1987. This laboratory has investigated the mechanisms of brain tumor growth and control for almost twenty years. Early on, it described the importance of growth factors in brain tumor development and assessed the central role of angiogenesis in these tumors; recently it has begun to use this knowledge to develop targeted therapies such as Gleevec and anti-angiogenic therapies to treat brain tumors. It has also been involved in imaging tumors to do molecular neurosurgery. Because this laboratory is in the Department of Neurosurgery, it is particularly interested in the use of local therapies for tumors. These therapies include the ability to leave slow-release polymers in the tumor bed, to put stem cells in the tumor bed that will track down tumor cells, and to infuse anti-tumor molecules directly into the tumor.

The Black Laboratory is part of a larger Brigham and Women's Neurosurgical Oncology Laboratory that includes molecular analysis of brain tumors, a study of immunology, and advanced work in brain tumor imaging. In turn, the Neurosurgical Oncology Laboratory participates in the Dana-Farber/Harvard Cancer Center Neuro-Oncology Program. This program includes BWH clinical researchers: in neuro-oncology, Dr. Patrick Wen, Dr. Santosh Kesari, and Dr. Jan Drappatz; in radiology, Dr. Alexandra Golby, Dr. Peter Black, Dr. Ron Kikinis, and Dr. Ferenc Jolesz; in neuropathology, Dr. Rebecca Folkerth, Dr. Keith Ligon, and Dr. Jennifer Chen; in basic biology, Dr. Charles Stiles and Dr. Ron DePinho; and in translational research, Dr. Mark Johnson, Dr. Rona Carroll, Dr. Arnab Chakravarti, and myself. This group of dedicated scientists gives some idea of the depth and breadth of brain tumor research at one institution and is a mini-example of how this work is organized.

The exciting research noted in this chapter is one of the major reasons to be hopeful about the treatment of your brain tumor. In the next chapter, you will find a guide to some of the more conventional drugs that are often prescribed to help control some of the conditions associated with brain tumors and their therapies.

15

———■———

Drugs for Swelling, Seizures,
and Other Problems

Research is keeping us on the cutting-edge of new developments for treating brain tumors, and existent techniques allow doctors to provide an impressive array of options for care. Daunting though it may be, the reality for a brain tumor patient is that treating the tumor is only part of the story. Too often the course of a patient's life has been changed by a seizure at work that demonstrated to all her colleagues that she was different, or changed by the effects of steroids that make the face obese and weaken the muscles.

Many attendant medications are part of the daily life of a patient with a brain tumor. Many patients, for example, take steroids to control swelling and anticonvulsants to control seizures. Your doctor may also prescribe pain medication and anti-emetics (to control vomiting). In this chapter, I will explain why these drugs are prescribed, which types are appropriate for different types of brain tumors, and what kinds of side effects you can expect when you take these medications.

Many of these drugs have similar names, and it's easy to get confused about which is which. All drugs also have two names: a generic (general) name and a trade name. In this chapter and throughout the book, the generic name will come first, followed by the trade name (it will be capitalized) in parentheses. Unpatented drugs are known by their protocol numbers rather than by generic and trade names.

Ask your doctor for clear, written instructions and a schedule of when you should take these medications and how much you should take. Buy an inexpensive plastic box at the pharmacy to help you keep track of your drugs and their dosage schedule; if you tend to forget whether you have taken a medication, have someone in your family take the responsibility of giving your medications to you. If you have questions about the timing of a medication or about what to do if you miss a dose, call your nurse or doctor.

You may also wish to purchase a copy of the *Physician's Desk Reference* (PDR), a large book, published annually, that contains useful information about the dosages and side effects of most drugs. Often Googling a drug name on the Internet will also give you important information, but be careful about the sources of this information.

Terms You May Hear: Drugs for Swelling, Seizures, and Other Problems

Bolus: A concentrated drug or contrast medium (for a diagnostic scan) injected into a blood vessel or given intravenously.

Controlled-release capsule: Drugs released slowly over a period of time.

Dose rate: The amount of medication given over a certain period of time; for example, 5 cc per hour.

Enteral: Medicine that is given by mouth in either solid or liquid form.

Parenteral: Medicine that is delivered in such a way that it bypasses the intestines; usually administered through the veins or into the skin or muscle, rather than through the mouth.

Corticosteroids

What they're for: Glucocorticosteroids, or steroids for short, help to control swelling in the brain. These drugs, which are synthetic forms of the steroid hormones that our adrenal glands produce, have revolutionized the way in which we manage disorders that create significant swelling in the brain. Brain swelling can produce major problems with weakness, sensory loss, or speech difficulty.

What they are called:

- dexamethasone (Decadron; also Aeroseb-Dex, Alba-Dex, Decaderm, Decadrol, Decasone R.p., Decaspray, Deenar, Deronil, Dex-4, Dexace, Dexameth, Dezone, Gammacorten, Hexadrol, Maxidex)
- methylprednisolone (Medrol; also Depo-Medrol, Medlone 21, Meprolone, Metrocort, Metypred, Solu-Medrol, Summicort)
- prednisone (Delta-Dome, Deltasone, Liquid Pred, Lisacort, Meticorten, Orasone, Prednicen-M, Sk-Prednisone, Sterapred)

Abbreviations on Your Containers of Medicine

The following abbreviations may show up on your prescription labels or in written instructions from your doctor.

i, ii, iii	one, two, three
Q	every; for example, Q 4 H = every four hours
QD	every day
BID	twice a day
TID	three times a day
QID	four times a day
PO	by mouth
IV	intravenous
IM	intramuscular

What you should know about them: Steroids can be helpful, but they also can interact poorly with other drugs you may be taking to control seizures, infections, or pain. Be sure to let the prescribing physician know about every other drug you are taking, including birth control pills, hormone replacement therapy, diet drugs, and diuretics.

While you are taking steroids, your immune system will not be as effective as usual. Stay away from children or adults who have recently been vaccinated against measles or polio or have received any other vaccines that contain a live virus.

Tell your health care team about any side effects you experience.

When you take synthetic steroids, especially if you have been taking them for a while, your body may stop secreting a natural steroid called cortisol. You will need to stop taking synthetic steroids gradually (this is called tapering off) so that your adrenal glands can resume their role as manufacturers of the steroids that your body needs. Suddenly stopping your intake of synthetic steroids altogether can be very dangerous.

As with any drug, follow your doctor's directions for taking steroids. *Never stop taking them without consulting him or her first. You may become extremely weak and even die from not having enough steroid if your body has gotten used to this medication.*

Side Effects

The long-term use of steroids can lead to many side effects, so follow directions for their dosing carefully, and contact your health care team if you have any questions or concerns.

- Weight gain and water retention. "I felt like the Michelin man. I couldn't tie my shoes," one patient said.
- Swelling in the legs, face, and abdomen
- A bump below your neck, between the shoulders
- Sleeplessness, jumpiness
- Upset stomach, ulcers caused by increased production of stomach acid
- Muscle aches and weakness (myopathy)
- Hair growth on the face
- Skin changes (acne and stretch marks on your mid-section and legs)
- Mood swings, anxiety
- Risk of infection
- Risk of blood clots in the legs

Less common side effects include:

- Osteoporosis
- Diabetes mellitus
- Eye cataracts

Despite these side effects, steroids may sometimes make the difference between suffering a terrible disability from having a brain tumor and living a quite tolerable life.

Anticonvulsants

What they're for: Anticonvulsants, or antiepileptic drugs, can help prevent seizures or convulsions. They work by reducing the electrical signals in the brain that can trigger a seizure. Brain tumors are particularly irritating to the brain and have a high tendency to cause seizures (see chapter 2).
What they are called:

- diphenylhydantoin/phenytoin (Dilantin; also Cerebyx, Mesantoin, Peganone, Phenytex)

This anticonvulsant is often given in the hospital before or after surgery to control seizures. Some people are allergic to Dilantin; it may cause a rash that looks like measles over the body. If you develop this rash, do not stop taking this drug by yourself, but notify your doctor. He or she will most likely give you another anti-seizure medication. The rash will usually go away within a week after you stop taking Dilantin. You should not take this drug if you are pregnant because of the slight risk of birth defects. Also, good dental care is important while you are taking Dilantin because the gums tend to hypertrophy. Rarely, it may change the blood count in the body.

- carbamazepine (Tegretal; also Atreto, Epitol, Tegretol)

Tegretol is a good alternative to Dilantin and is often prescribed to prevent generalized seizures. It may produce a rash, lowering of the white blood count, drowsiness, and jaundice.

- valproate; valproic acid (Depakote, Depkene)

This drug may also be prescribed for tonic-clonic seizures (those that cause jerking motions of the arms and legs). It is well tolerated but can cause liver toxicity, so careful monitoring of liver function tests is necessary. This drug can also affect the white blood cells and platelets, so they should also be monitored.

- phenobarbital—may be prescribed as an anticonvulsant for children or for adults who cannot tolerate other drugs; sedating, and therefore is less used now that alternatives are available.
- lorazepam (Ativan)—short-acting drug taken under the tongue (sublingually) or intravenously to lessen or prevent seizures. It is the treatment of choice for *status epilepticus,* a condition in which there is continuous seizure activity.
- diazepam (Valium)—short-acting anticonvulsant that also may be used for status epilepticus. It is not used as often as some of the other anticonvulsants because of its risks of cardiac arrest and respiratory depression.
- levetiracetam (Keppra)—increasingly popular as an alternative to Dilantin.

Other less commonly used anti-seizure medications include trileptal, lamictal, zonegran, neurontin, topamax, and klonopin. These drugs may be just as effective as those listed above, and it may be worth trying several drugs until one works.

What you should know about them: Carefully follow your doctor's advice about taking these drugs, and do not stop taking them unless you've checked with the doctor first. Be sure to tell your doctor if you are taking any other medications while you are taking anti-convulsants. They can make some chemotherapy drugs less effective.

Your blood levels will need to be monitored often while you are taking anti-seizure medication to make sure you are taking the right amount. Dilantin, Tegretol, phenobarbital, trileptal, and Depakote are all monitored with levels drawn from the blood, and each individual's dose may differ depending on the level. Other anti-seizure medications are dose-dependent; they do not require blood levels to be drawn.

Alcohol can decrease the effectiveness of this kind of medication, and some foods and medicines, such as some antacids (Tums or Maalox), anti-depressants, corticosteroids, and antibiotics, can interfere with metabolism.

Side Effects
- Rash (with Dilantin)
- Dizziness (with Dilantin)

- Constipation (with Dilantin)
- Trouble with balance (with Dilantin)
- Facial hair (with Dilantin)
- Thickening of the gums (with Dilantin)
- Headaches
- Tiredness (with Dilantin, phenobarbital, Keppra)
- Sensitivity to the sun (Tegretol)
- Infection (with Tegretol)

Rare but serious side effects of Dilantin include a type of anemia called aplastic anemia, and other blood abnormalities.

Pain Medicines (Analgesics)

What they're for: Although the brain itself does not feel pain, if you have a brain tumor you may experience headaches, soreness around a surgical suture, and other types of discomfort.

What they are called: Medicines for pain relief include analgesics, non-steroidal anti-inflammatory agents, and opioid narcotics. Talk with your health care team about which type of medication is best for you. Some hospitals also have a pain team that can consult with you about pain management.

- acetaminophen (Tylenol)—This mild pain reliever can also reduce fever, but it does not generally enhance bleeding as aspirin does— thus it is often used instead of aspirin. Acetaminophen is analgesic (it alleviates pain), but has little anti-inflammatory action.
- Darvocet, Darvon—These combination drugs include a strong pain reliever with Tylenol (Darvocet) or aspirin (Darvon).
- non-steroidal anti-inflammatory drugs (NSAIDs): ibuprofen (Advil, Motrin); toridol—These drugs control pain, fever, and inflammation and are often associated with stomach irritation. NSAIDs should be avoided or used sparingly during chemotherapy, because they can decrease the body's production of platelets.
- codeine—a narcotic that has substantial effects on the bowel, causing constipation and nausea.

- opiates: morphine, controlled-release morphine (MS Contin, Oramorph), methadone, meperidine (Demerol), oxycodone (Oxycontin, Roxicodone in Percocet, Percodan, which contains aspirin)—These strong analgesics can change and slow respiration. They also have a substantial risk of addiction.

What you should know about them: You may take pain medication orally, through an IV, or through a patch. Some of my patients are concerned about becoming addicted to narcotics that they take for the pain related to a brain tumor, but this does not happen very often if these medications are taken for a short time only.

Side Effects
- **NSAIDs:** Stomach irritation is an important side effect and may require antacids and medications that diminish the production of stomach acid.
- **narcotics:** Morphine and meperidine (Demerol) can have a sedative effect that may make you tired and slow your breathing down. A drug called naloxone (Narcan) reverses the narcotic effect and may help. Narcotics may also cause your body to make histamine that can cause a rash. A medicine called diphenhydramine (Benadryl) can usually take care of that. Last, narcotics may make you constipated. We tell our patients to drink plenty of fluids. Sometimes docusate (Colace), a stool softener, is helpful.

Antipyretics

Antipyretics are drugs used to lower fever. Acetaminophen (Tylenol) and aspirin are the most common.

Antibiotics

What they're for: These infection-fighting medications may be important for patients who have had brain surgery. They are given on a preventive basis (prophylactically) for most surgery and may be needed if there is a question of infection.

Oxacillin and Nafcillin are intravenous agents that combat *Staphylococcus* infections, which are often the cause of wound and shunt infections. The emergence of strains of *Staphylococcus* that resist these drugs is an important feature of modern medicine—for these strains vancomycin must be used.

- Dicloxacillin is taken by mouth to fight *Staphylococcus.*
- Vancomycin is useful for treating infections caused by *S. aureus* and *S. epidermi*, especially if these are methicillin-resistant *staphylococcus aureus* bacteria (MRSA).
- cefazolin (Ancef), a so-called first-generation cephalosporin, is another good drug for fighting staph infections as well as gram-negative organisms.

What you should know about them: Antibiotics should be used only for bacteria that are known to be sensitive to them—sensitivity testing is an important prerequisite for choosing the right drug for a given situation. Antibiotics may select out bacteria that are resistant to them, so that it becomes harder and harder to eradicate the bacteria in your body. Your physician will prescribe antibiotics with care, because ultimately you may get fungal or other superinfections that are difficult to destroy.

Side effects: Antibiotics may produce a rash—they are the most likely drugs to cause a rash of unknown source. They may also produce diarrhea because they change the normal bacterial content of the bowel.

Anti-Emetics

What they're for: These drugs can keep nausea under control.

What they are called: A drug called odansetron (Zofran) is the most effective anti-emetic, but it is quite expensive. Another anti-emetic that is often used is promethazine (Phenergan).

Side effects: Anti-emetics may cause drowsiness, but this side effect is uncommon.

Mannitol and Furosemide

Mannitol (Osmotrol) may sometimes be given in the hospital to reduce cerebral swelling or relieve intracranial pressure. It works by drawing water out of the brain tissue. This drug is also given before some forms of chemotherapy to disrupt the blood-brain barrier, allowing the chemotherapeutic drug to enter the brain.

Furosemide (Lasix), a diuretic, causes excretion of water by the kidneys. It may be combined with mannitol to diminish the amount of fluid in the body generally.

Many drugs can help make the quality of life better for patients with brain tumors even if they do not primarily treat the tumor. In the next chapter, I will describe situations in which some patients decide to take these medicines for supportive care only; that is, they choose to forgo treatment of the tumor itself.

16

—■—

Choosing Supportive Care

At some time in the course of a malignant brain tumor, it is likely that treatment options will run out. In that case, supportive care—meaning care that focuses on making a patient comfortable when no active therapy can improve his or her condition—may be the only possible option. Here are the stories of two families that demonstrate the complexity of this decision.

Charles and Melissa MacKinnon

Charles MacKinnon was a successful defense attorney. At the age of fifty-six, this tall, confident man had reached the peak of his profession. He was a well-respected member of the bar. His wife, Melissa, and their four children enjoyed sailing off Cape Cod in the summer. In every sense, he was enjoying the prime of his life.

Charles had a significant past medical history. Seven years ago, Melissa had noticed that Charles was having occasional trouble speaking. In the courtroom, where he usually felt energized by rapid-fire exchanges with witnesses and prosecutors, he occasionally became anxious and hesitated as he struggled to find the right word. He went to see his primary care physician, who immediately sent Charles for a magnetic resonance scan. It showed what appeared to be a low-grade glioma. Charles and Melissa went home and searched the Internet for everything they could find about gliomas. They learned that most gliomas are removed surgically, but the outcome of surgery varies depending on the patient's age and degree of disability. They talked with a friend whose brother had had a brain tumor about where to go for treatment and checked on which surgeons had extensive experience with these tumors.

They came to see me one morning in March. After taking Charles's history, doing a neurological examination, and reviewing his scans, I explained the procedure to remove the tumor and asked if they had any questions. Charles was most concerned about impairment after surgery and the outlook for his health over the next five years. "If I'm going to be seriously disabled, I'd rather die," he said. I told him that he would most likely be facing increasing disability if the tumor continued to grow.

Two weeks later, I removed about 70 percent of Charles's tumor using awake surgery with brain mapping in the intraoperative MRI (see chapter 11). Thirty percent of the tumor was intermixed with nerve cells that were essential for speech and could not be removed. He had no speech deficit after surgery and not long afterward returned to the active practice of law.

For seven years, Charles did extremely well, maintaining his active law practice. Earlier this past year, however, he began to have difficulty speaking again. A new MRI scan revealed a mass that appeared to be a recurrent tumor. It was larger than the first and now showed up with the contrast (dye) that was used with the test. This tumor had appeared since his last checkup three months before. We did a PET scan that confirmed that this new tumor was probably malignant. I presented Charles's story and images to our tumor board, which meets weekly. It is made up of neurosurgeons, neuroradiologists, neuropathologists, neuro-oncologists, and radiation oncologists. We reviewed Charles's history and looked at his scan together. We unanimously recommended surgery to remove the new mass.

I told the MacKinnons about the board's suggestion and advised them that another operation was probably the best option, even though he might have more speaking trouble. With or without surgery, he would most likely have to stop practicing law altogether. Charles and Melissa went home to tell their children and prepare for the operation.

Two days before the scheduled operation, Melissa came to my office to ask me more questions about possible surgical outcomes. What exactly was his quality of life going to be like? Would he have pain? How long would he live? Were any new treatments needed for his care? What were the chances of complications from the surgery?

I told her that we would take some of the tumor out, but because of its aggressive nature, it almost certainly would come back, causing headaches and increasing speech difficulties. I said that the operation did have risks, though it was impossible to predict the exact outcome or how much more time Charles would have with or without the operation.

Later that day, Melissa called to say that she and Charles had decided not to proceed with the operation and wished to stop treatment altogether. He didn't want the rest of his life to be spent in continued chemotherapy and radiation. Melissa asked if he could have intravenous morphine at home in increasing doses to control his suffering. I told her that we could give him other forms of pain relief and recommended some medicines that he could take by mouth.

Charles gave up his law practice, his speech worsened, and a month later, he developed greater weakness on his right side. Melissa spent most of her time taking care of him. They spent many hours together. Three months later, he died at home.

Francine and Ellen

Francine, a seventy-eight-year-old woman from Providence, Rhode Island, was a retired nurse. When Francine's husband died several years ago, her daughter Ellen moved in with her. They were very devout Catholics who began every morning with mass at the church down the block from where they lived.

Ellen brought Francine to a hospital two years ago when she was experiencing weakness, confusion, memory loss, and sleepiness. Ellen thought that her mother may have had a stroke. Instead, an MRI showed that she had a probable glioblastoma. Francine's doctor recommended that she come to the Brigham and Women's Hospital in Boston for treatment.

Over the next year, in spite of surgery, radiation therapy, three kinds of chemotherapy, and focused radiation, her tumor spread throughout much of her brain. She couldn't speak and was so weak she could not get out of bed. Her right side was immobilized, and we had to give her blood thinners to prevent blood clots from traveling to her lungs.

One night, I was called to see Francine at 11 P.M. Her condition had suddenly deteriorated and she was comatose. A CT scan showed bleeding into her tumor. Ellen was sleeping in a chair beside Francine's bed, and woke up when I came into the room. I talked with her about what had happened and told her that there really were no good options for her mother. At best, we could only keep Francine comfortable.

Ellen, who appeared to be about fifty years old and who was usually mild mannered, became angry and direct. She asked, in fact, demanded, that we take the blood clot out, although I told her that the chance of Francine surviving more than three months after it was removed was very small and that she could continue to bleed because of her blood thinners. Ellen was adamantly convinced that there would be a miracle and wanted "everything that can possibly be done." She reminded me that her mother had named her proxy in health care. Reluctantly, we operated and she improved slightly for three weeks. After that, however, she steadily deteriorated and in two months she died. She had not really been interactive since a point one week before her surgery.

These two patients illustrate the problem we are regularly faced with as surgeons: what to do about withdrawing treatment. In Charles's case, his own strong opinion, which was shared by his wife, led to the decision to withdraw treatment. An operation to remove his new aggressive tumor may have afforded him more time, but only with the potential for a compromised quality of life. In Francine's case, her proxy decision led to continued treatment where otherwise I would probably have stopped it.

How do doctors and patients make decisions about whether or not to continue fighting a brain tumor? Is it purely a matter of personal preference or are there some objective rules? If you have a brain tumor, where can you find guidance to help you decide?

Brain Death

A rare condition that should not be confused with the terminal condition we have been talking about thus far is brain death. Brain death is not a condition in which decisions have to be made about withdrawing care. It is death, and patients who fulfill certain specified criteria for this condition are considered to be dead. These criteria include lack of brain stem responses and lack of breathing, eye movements, and some reflexes. This condition can be satisfactorily diagnosed by modern neurologists and neurosurgeons and should lead to immediate cessation of support in most cases, as the patient is dead.

I tell my patients that we can pursue the most aggressive treatments, but if these procedures or drugs are going to harm them or not extend their life or quality of life, we should stop them. Even after we stop treating the tumor, we can continue to treat symptoms to improve a person's quality of life. Care continues even when medical options have been exhausted.

Although the decision to provide comfort measures only may seem impossible to make, there are well-accepted guidelines for this. I like to think of these guidelines as being based on the answers to five important questions:

1. What is the natural progression of the disease?
2. What are the likely side effects or consequences of treatment?
3. What are the available options for stopping treatment?
4. What do you and your family want to do?
5. What kinds of therapies will your insurance carrier allow?

Let's look at these questions in sequence.

Some Factors to Consider

1. What Is the Natural Progression of the Disease?

For many brain tumors, the course of the disease is now quite clear. For glioblastoma multiforme, a highly malignant brain tumor, the average survival after discovery is approximately nine to eighteen months depending on age and some other factors, which I discussed in chapter 4. In contrast, low-grade gliomas have differing survival rates, which are much longer. Patients with tumors like meningiomas or pituitary adenomas often have normal life spans.

Your doctor can usually give you an honest assessment of your prognosis. You can also learn more about the type of tumor you have and its impact on quality of life by talking with other patients who have shared the same diagnosis. Your neurosurgeon can ask a patient who has faced the same decision about treatment whether he or she would be willing to talk with you. Some hospitals have formal networks of patient support groups.

Regardless of the most likely course of the disease, the quality of remaining life is as important as the duration of that life. Patients who have tumors in the movement area of the brain or in the speech area may be absolutely miserable, although they're not necessarily about to die imminently. It is difficult for any one other than the patient to evaluate quality of life, but it does need to be factored in to the decision making.

2. What Are the Likely Side Effects or Consequences of Treatment?

The second important factor to consider in deciding whether or not to treat a brain tumor is the effect of the intervention. Is it likely to prolong life significantly? Is it going to add major risks or potential complications? Are there further treatments that need to be looked at? Answers to these questions are probabilities rather than certainties, but they are important to introduce into the decision-making process. Again, your doctor, family members, and other patients who have had this type of intervention can help you consider this important question.

3. What Are the Available Options for Stopping Treatment?

The third consideration involves the options for stopping treatment. A range of possibilities exists for patients who wish to stop aggressive interventions and allow the disease to take its course. They include the decision not to operate (the choice that Melissa and Charles made), and, at the end of life, the decision not to intubate or resuscitate, to withhold food and water, or to actively give morphine.

If you are in a hospital, the nurses or ethics committee may help you make these decisions. A do not rescuscitate/do not intubate (DNR/DNI) order can be readily written if you and your family wish it. The decision to withhold food and water is usually made by your surrogate decision maker when you are unable to decide for yourself. Morphine may be appropriate in the very late stages where pain is an important aspect of the tumor's effect.

As you review these options it is important to remember that, in most cases, you can change your mind about them. You can ask doctors not to insert a breathing tube, but change your mind and request one three days later if you wish. Living wills allow a patient to specify what kinds of states a patient does not want, but they do not have to say in detail what needs to be done. There is no way to predict with certainty how a person's disease will progress or how he or she will feel about further treatment at any given point. Sometimes a patient who has lived with a tumor that has been considered inoperable may begin to have more and more problems because of it. At that point, it's not too late to consider surgery as an option in order to stabilize the person enough so that he or she can have a better quality of life. At other times, as one of our nurses once said, "People think that they've come to the last chapter and in fact they continue on to the sequel."

Here are some of the options in supportive care:

Choosing not to treat with antibiotics. One way of choosing not to treat a brain tumor is to choose not to use antibiotics to fight pneumonia or a urinary tract infection. The likely result of this choice is that infection will ultimately cause death, but this may take many weeks.

Choosing not to resuscitate. Choosing "not to resuscitate" means that if there should be spontaneous cardiac arrest, the medical team would not use the usual techniques for restoring a heartbeat. These techniques include calling the code team, putting a breathing tube in the lung (intubation), external chest compression or direct heart massage to start the heart, and injection of epinephrine into the heart. These are all aggressive and invasive techniques that are part of the usual response to a heart arrest in the modern hospital.

Choosing to withdraw a breathing tube. Extubation, or removing a breathing tube when a patient is at least partly dependent on the ventilator, is another way of hastening death.

Our thinking has changed considerably in deciding what is possible with patients who are terminally ill. For example, there used to be a distinction between stopping treatment and not starting it. Doctors often thought that they would feel more comfortable not putting a tube in a patient to help him or her breathe than in taking it out.

These distinctions, which seem to have little moral significance, have been less important in recent times. There is an increasing acceptance of the concept that passive withdrawal of care with an intention to shorten life is essentially the same as more active seeking of death. Withholding food and water, for example, was once considered drastic and inappropriate. It is now a well-accepted course of treatment under the right circumstance.

Choosing to withdraw a feeding tube. The courts have recently accepted the decision to withdraw a feeding tube as an acceptable treatment decision hastening death. The reason for this decision is that feeding by a tube in a terminal condition is extraordinary and may not be warranted. Whatever the reason, a family or surrogate decision maker can ask that the feeding tube be withdrawn.

Choosing to give increasing doses of morphine. Morphine, a powerful narcotic, is often given for pain relief to patients with end-stage disease. It may also slow the patient's breathing.

When Melissa asked me to give this drug to Charles, I refused because his disease, though painful, had not progressed to the point at which we considered his status to be terminal. However, in a hospitalized patient who has intractable pain, increasing amounts of morphine may be necessary. This administration brings in the "doctrine of the double effect" in medical ethics. This doctrine suggests that a treatment that might not be allowed by itself (that is, giving morphine to stop a patient's breathing) might nevertheless be used if its primary intention were to relieve pain.

What Do You Want to Do? A generation ago, the decision to withdraw or not to proceed with treatment would be left in large part to the physicians involved in the patient's care. The decision would be based on whether the treatment might work and on what seemed most appropriate for the patient. Recently this process has been changed to include more input from you (the patient) and your family. Eventually the decision-making process changed from what the doctor wanted to what you might think or want.

This view has been accepted legally and in most moral discussions so that the focus is now solely on the patient. If you are the patient, what do you want to do? If you are mentally competent, you can make the decision alone without input from your physicians or family. If you are a Jehovah's Witness, you can refuse to have a blood transfusion. If you have a life-threatening condition that would benefit from surgery or other major interventions, you can refuse to have such therapies even if they have a strong likelihood of helping. The trend that has emerged in America is an extension of the belief in autonomy and self-direction of our lives: you as a patient get to decide what happens to you.

How can you ensure that your choices about treatment will be followed if you become mentally incompetent or comatose? There are two well-recognized ways to make sure that your wishes are respected. One is to use a document called an advance directive or living will (see the Appendix) to make your wishes clear so that doctors and others will know what they should do. The second approach is to pick someone who will be your spokesperson—a health care proxy (see the Appendix) who can speak for you about important decisions. Although Francine did not have a living will on file at the hospital, she had signed a form that listed Ellen as her health care proxy.

If your doctor or nurse suggests that you put together a will and health care proxy, don't assume that he or she has given up hope for you. Rather, it's a good idea for all individuals to have these forms in place so that family members aren't burdened with decisions without some input from the person who is ill.

4. What Does Your Family Want to Do?

As you weigh the decision about whether or not to treat your brain tumor, you most likely will turn to your family for support and advice. The decision, as I noted earlier, is influenced by several factors that are disease driven: for instance, the decision to undergo surgery for one type of tumor that most likely will not recur is quite different than the decision to undergo surgery for a tumor that, like Charles's, probably would return and create further impairment. In addition to these disease-driven factors, there are personal factors. A young mother with two dependent children may be less willing to undergo risky procedures than a single person who is further along in life.

Likewise, the opinions of family members can vary dramatically from patient to patient. If you find that your decision about whether or not to treat your tumor is at odds with what your loved one feels is best for you, you may wish to talk with a social worker or a member of the ethics committee at your hospital for some suggestions about how to come to a resolution.

These resources also may be called into play for patients who are children, especially if the child's parents and physicians do not see eye to eye on the best course of treatment. Parents can choose not to treat a brain tumor in their child, but if the hospital feels that such an operation may be lifesaving and in the child's best interest, the legal office of the hospital may get involved. In some cases, hospitals have even applied to take guardianship of the child from the parents in order to pursue treatment.

5. What Kinds of Therapies Will Your Insurance Carrier Allow?

Recently, another voice has emerged in the decision-making process along with the doctors, the family, and the patient. This is the voice of the insurance company. Some insurance companies, for example, will not pay for expensive chemotherapies that do not have a high likelihood of improving care, and very few will pay for experimental therapies, which often are the appropriate treatment for advanced tumors.

Policies vary from carrier to carrier and from state to state. In some states, the lack of insurance support for lifesaving treatments has become a public policy concern. Bills that would mandate insurance coverage for brain tumor treatment are under consideration.

If your neurosurgeon recommends a particular therapy that is not covered by your insurance plan, you should find out if an experimental protocol is available (see chapter 14).

Additional Resources to Help You Decide

If you are trying to decide whether to start or stop treatment for your brain tumor, talk with your doctor and your family about the factors to consider. Weigh the likely difference in outcome between treating and not treating, the effects of the treatment, and most important, what *you* want. You may also want to take advantage of the following resources within the hospital to help you make this decision.

Chaplaincy Services

Most hospitals now offer chaplaincy services. A minister, priest, rabbi, or other spiritual leader can be a useful resource, especially if you have strong religious beliefs. Knowing what the options are will be very important. Each religious tradition has its own approach to such decisions. Whether you are a devout practitioner of your faith or someone for whom religion has been unimportant, you may wish to talk with a clergy member to explore your feelings about this important decision.

Hospital Ethics Committees

Most hospitals now have ethics committees composed of nurses, doctors, attorneys, clergy, and laypersons. These committees consult with patients and their families to help evaluate the situation and establish that the withdrawal or the continuation of treatment is appropriate. Often they can be extremely useful in helping families recognize when treatment may be futile. They can provide clarity, comfort, and support.

Ethics committees can also be helpful if a patient does not have a living will and his or her family appears to be making decisions that the doctor or hospital has reason to believe the patient would not want. In most hospitals, they can be asked to consult by the nurses or doctors taking care of you.

Social Workers, Psychologists, and Psychiatrists

Personal help from a social worker, psychologist, or psychiatrist may be an important element in getting through the crisis of care. Ellen Golden, a social worker at our hospital, says that people who have chosen to stop treating a brain tumor may experience a wide range of emotions, from relief and gratefulness to sadness and grief. Friends and family members will respond to your decision with loving support, but it is not uncommon to feel blame from those who think you have "given up" and are "giving in to the tumor." Golden says, "People may ask, 'Why don't you go somewhere and try a clinical trial? Why aren't you fighting to the end? You never know unless you try.'"

Golden talks with patients about being able to say, "I'm not pursuing treatment, because it's not about finding a cure now, it's about finding care that will enhance my quality of life: spending time with my friends and family out of the hospital and not having my life dictated by medicine that doesn't make me feel good. I don't want to add any more side effects to what I'm already coping with. I don't want to die and I want to be here as long as I can, but if being here as long as I can means traveling around the country and feeling sick, that's not what I choose. I choose to be at home with my family. It's about doing things that are important to me now and not letting the tumor dictate how I'm going to live my life."

It's important to feel good about your decision and to let people know how you arrived at it and what it means for you. In many cases it doesn't necessarily mean that your life is over. In brain tumor support groups, Golden says, we sometimes see two people with the same type of tumor; one has elected to pursue surgery, radiation, and chemotherapy; the other has chosen to wait and see if the tumor progresses. Some patients choose not to pursue treatment out of a sense of denial about the tumor. They may think, "Maybe they're wrong. Why take these risks associated with treatment? I don't want to put my family through this and my insurance won't cover it."

If you are struggling with a range of emotions and feelings of guilt about "giving up" and letting people down, talking with a social worker, priest, psychiatrist, or friend can help. A counselor can talk with you about your struggle to balance your decision with your family and friends' insistence that you keep fighting. You may be able to express your desire to be alive and healthy with and for those you love, as well as your realization that you have fought enough. Now you simply want to be with them as well and as long as you can.

Hospice Care

When we left the rehabilitation hospital, we called on hospice to help with our care of Tina at home. They provided nursing care and took over the ordering of drugs. The nurse came twice a week. The nursing assistant came three times a week to help in keeping Tina clean and comfortable. At first the assistant was coming every day. It proved to be too much for Tina and for us. We asked that she come less frequently.
—John Hammock, *An Open Approach to Living with Cancer*

If you choose to receive hospice care—that is, skilled nursing care at home—in order to obtain insurance coverage, your physician will have to certify in writing that your diagnosis may limit your life to less than six months. However, you can go on and off hospice care, and beginning hospice does not mean that you have to end your relationship with your other health care providers. In fact, you can still return to the hospital if you change your mind about being cared for at home. You can also return to receive radiation therapy or medication to alleviate pain and maximize the quality of your life.

At this time, psychiatrist Malcolm Rogers says, your family may wish to have a direct conversation with your physician about what to expect in the days and weeks ahead. "When people perceive that someone is not going to recover," Rogers suggests "[t]hey need acknowledgement of that. Having some expectation of what will happen makes it easier. Our culture doesn't expose us to dying and death. Families need to know that the comfort measures of hospice care are there to minimize suffering. Also, most people who are dying of brain tumors have some gradual loss in their awareness of what's happening, and so they are not suffering."

Although every situation is unique, the health care team can help families know what to expect in terms of the symptoms and signs that will occur, how quickly the process will be, and whether it will be painful. A mental health professional such as a social worker, psychologist, or psychiatrist can also help families as well as the patient, who may fear pain, loss of control, and being left alone. It may help to consider that often when a person with a brain tumor is nearing the end of his life, he is less afraid than he was early on, when the brain tumor was diagnosed.

Symptoms that we often see at this stage are difficulties with speech and swallowing, lethargy, incontinence, and difficulty with walking. A person may become increasingly drowsy or lapse into a coma.

Families can help at this time by turning and moving their bedridden loved one frequently to prevent bedsores. They can provide ice chips and swab their loved one's face and lips. At the end of life, patients often lose their appetite, but they do not suffer because of this.

In the very last days, the person's breathing may be labored, but in this phase she will be unconscious, so he or she will not be afraid. Often a person's transition to death is peaceful.

Families want to do whatever they can to help their loved one in the last days or weeks, but often the greatest thing they can do is to simply be with their loved one. Even at the end of life, Rogers says, patients and families can hope, and this is not an empty hope. He adds, "The thing that redeems this is an intimacy within families that occurs. This intimacy is kind of unique, and these special moments within families are often very positive."

Decisions not to treat brain tumors are always difficult, but they are increasingly acceptable in medical institutions today. Withdrawing treatment is as acceptable as not treating from the beginning. In each case, the disease itself, the effectiveness of the proposed treatment, the available options, and the patient's wishes are all considered carefully in an effort to surmount the many challenges and doubts surrounding this type of choice and, finally, to come to a decision with which the patient is comfortable.

Now that we have reviewed the spectrum of treatment options for adults, let's explore the options that are available for the treatment of brain tumors in children. Then we will describe some of the resources that are available to add to a person's quality of life while fighting a tumor. These resources include counseling, support groups, and integrative therapies like acupuncture and massage.

17

—◼—

Treatment of Brain Tumors
in Children

The brain tumors that affect children are quite different than those in adults. They include medulloblastomas in the cerebellum; ependymomas in the fourth ventricle; gliomas in the brain stem and thalamus; cranio-pharyngiomas in the suprasellar space (near the pituitary gland); and primitive neuroectodermal tumors and dysplastic neuroepithelial tumors in the cerebral hemispheres. You may wish to turn back to chapter 1 for an overview of these varieties of tumors and their locations.

Medulloblastomas, the most common malignant pediatric tumors, arise in the cerebellum and sometimes spread throughout the nervous system. *Gliomas* occur in children as well as adults, but they can have a different pattern, depending on their location. These tumors include diffuse brain stem gliomas, which are malignant and difficult to treat; optic system gliomas, which may be part of a disorder called neurofibromatosis; pilocytic astrocytomas of the cerebellum, which may be cured with surgery; and cerebral hemisphere gliomas, which have varying patterns.

Some pediatric tumors can be cured; these include the pilocytic astrocytomas of the cerebellum, choroid plexus papillomas, and dysem-

---

Note: Members of the Pediatric Brain Tumor treatment team at Dana-Farber/Children's Hospital Cancer Center were particularly helpful in preparing this chapter.

bryoplastic neuroepithelial tumors (DNTs). Medulloblastomas and ger-
minomas also may be cured, despite being malignant tumors.

Whatever the tumor type or location, the most sophisticated care of a
child with a brain tumor is through a specialized pediatric neuro-
oncology group at a children's hospital.

Diagnosis

Head tilt, unsteadiness, headache, and vomiting are often early signs of a
childhood brain tumor, because many of these tumors in children are in
the cerebellum. Visual loss, double vision, and seizures are other symptoms to watch for. A child who is diagnosed with a brain tumor may go
from being well one day to being hospitalized the next. The child may have
some dizziness and a headache, which the parents may attribute to an ear
or sinus infection. If the headaches lead to vomiting, the pediatrician may
request a computed tomographic (CT) scan, and the results may land the
child and his parents in the hospital emergency room, in shock, faced with
an operation to remove a large tumor. Tish Reidy, a nurse practioner at
Children's Hospital in Boston, notes, "Just the word *tumor* is so scary.
Many children undergo brain surgery within twenty-four hours of their
diagnosis and the family has no time to process what's going on."

Occasionally, brain tumors in both adults and children are discovered
through scans taken for other reasons. A CT after a head injury may reveal
an apparent brain tumor that has not caused symptoms. Sometimes
removal of the tumor is the right treatment even if it is not producing
symptoms.

Christopher Turner, M.D., director of outcomes research for pediatric
neuro-oncology at the Dana-Farber/Children's Hospital Cancer Center in
Boston, says that it is best for these children to be taken to a center that
specializes in treating children with brain tumors. These centers exist
throughout the country (see Resources), and some are more comprehensive than others. Although many smaller centers can give chemotherapy,
if the child needs surgery, it is preferable to have it take place at a center
with a pediatric neurosurgeon. Often the support services that these
centers can provide (such as radiation departments with specialists who
have been trained in working with children, pediatric anesthesiologists,

neuro-oncology teams, and social services) cannot be found in local community hospitals. Just as for treatment of a brain tumor in an adult, it's best to find an entire team of specialists you are comfortable working with and who will be able to answer any and all questions to your satisfaction.

Dr. Mark Kieran, director of pediatric medical neuro-oncology at the Dana-Farber/Children's Hospital Cancer Center, points out that as you look at potential treatment centers, it's important to examine their "cure rates" carefully. Some centers emphasize the number of brain tumor survivors, but the quality of life for children who are living with brain tumors is also important. Look for a center with support systems that enable survivors to lead a good life after treatment. To take your child to such a place, you may need to travel some distance away from the support of friends and relatives. Consider a Ronald McDonald house or other charitable institution where you can stay and be fed at no charge, and, if possible, a place that is equipped with transportation to take you back and forth to the hospital.

Treatment

Parents usually want to know what they can do (such as change their child's diet) to help their child in addition to the treatment that he or she will receive at the hospital. Again, a lot of research still needs to be done about the best way to manage brain tumors in children, and many questions remain unanswered. Many children have an operation, leave the hospital, and then need ongoing treatment. Some children go on to have radiation therapy. Some have chemotherapy. Some need all three—surgery, radiation, and chemotherapy—and may require a year to a year and a half of intensive medical treatment.

Although more children are being cured of brain tumors than ever before, in order to cure the tumor, there is often a price to be paid. The consequences range from the side effects of surgery, radiation, and chemotherapy to physical changes in appearance, behavioral and personality changes, mild to severe memory loss, learning disabilities, seizures, slow growth, weight gain, or sterility.

Surgery

As with adults, surgery is often the first step in therapy for brain tumors in children. Your child's surgeon should make both you and your child feel comfortable, and he or she should have experience with pediatric brain tumors. For many brain tumors in children, surgery is the only necessary treatment. The child has surgery and is followed with regular checkups—nothing else needs to be done. In other cases, we combine surgery with radiation and chemotherapy. Some tumors are located in a part of brain where we can't operate, so we start these patients on a course of radiation and chemotherapy soon after diagnosis.

Emergency Surgery

Dr. Liliana Goumnerova, a pediatric neurosurgeon and director of clinical pediatric neurosurgical oncology at the Dana-Farber/Children's Hospital Cancer Center, notes that in many cases, surgery for brain tumors in children is performed on an urgent basis. The child may have seizures, headaches, or vomiting, and his family will take him to the emergency room where he will have a diagnostic scan and other tests. If a mass is found, the child will be admitted to the hospital so that he can have surgery right away.

The staff in the emergency room will send the child's blood sample to the hospital blood bank so that the surgical team will have blood on hand for a transfusion if necessary. The child's parents will meet with the anesthesiologist just before surgery. Then the neurosurgeon will oversee the child's care until after surgery, when the entire team of oncologists and other specialists will see the child.

Planned Surgery

If surgery is not an emergency, you will have more time to prepare your child and family.

The pre-operative visit (or visits). Although every hospital handles the pre-admissions process differently, in most centers, children who will undergo surgery to remove a brain tumor meet with an anesthesiologist from one week to one day before the operation. The child may also need multiple visits to the hospital to meet with various other specialists, such as an endocrinologist or an ophthalmologist. During this pre-operative period, the health care team is available by telephone to answer the parents' questions.

In contrast to a situation in which many trips to the hospital are required, at some centers the family visits a pre-operative clinic in the days before the operation. At this clinic, a single blood draw of a small amount can provide samples for blood cell counts, and for the hospital blood bank (in case a transfusion is necessary later). The family's meetings with specialists are coordinated in this clinic so that only one trip to the hospital is necessary. The health-care team assesses the child for recent developments in her health (for instance, does she have a cold?) as well as for other health problems (in addition to the brain tumor) for which she may need further testing or evaluation by specialists. At this time, the family also meets with a pediatric anesthesiologist and a nurse to answer any questions about the operation.

If the tumor is in the hypothalamic-pituitary region of the brain, and surgery is not needed on an emergency basis, the child may see an endocrinologist before the operation. Either the endocrinologist or an oncologist will do some baseline blood tests to begin monitoring the child for the development of hormonal deficiencies. In children, there is a limited period of time to treat disorders of growth; therefore, the earlier we recognize problems, the better off the child will be. This monitoring and surveillance for any problems in the child's growth and development will continue throughout treatment for the brain tumor and for many years into the future.

The day of surgery. On the day of your child's operation, you will bring him to the pre-operative area of the hospital. In most centers that treat children with brain tumors, other family members may accompany your child as well.

Talk with your spouse or partner ahead of time about how you will talk with your child as you turn him over to the surgical team. In some situations, one parent may be permitted to accompany the child while he has anesthesia induced. This is called a "parent present induction." Alternatively, a child may be heavily sedated in a pre-operative area immediately adjacent to the operating room so that the child is not frightened about leaving his parents.

A mother of a child with a brain tumor said that her husband stayed with their son while he was going under anesthesia because "he was strong when I wasn't strong." After his operation, they took turns staying with him in the hospital around-the-clock.

The point at which children are comfortable separating from their parents varies by age and developmental stage. Young infants, for instance, will not be concerned, whereas a three-year-old may be terrified and an adolescent may want his parents to leave quickly. Once the child is under anesthesia, he will be unconscious throughout surgery and oblivious to separation from his parents and discomfort.

Dr. Mark Rockoff, a pediatric anesthesiologist at Children's Hospital in Boston, encourages parents to ask questions and write them down ahead of time. He notes that there are many safe, comfortable ways to induce anesthesia in children, but not all methods are appropriate for all children, especially in emergency situations. Methods of accomplishing this vary according to the patient's age and disease. These include:

- *Oral sedatives,* which are commonly given to young children who may be frightened by needles. After the child swallows the sedative and gets sleepy, the anesthesiologist inserts an intravenous (IV) catheter or administers additional anesthesia via a mask.
- *Liquid medication may be given rectally* to a young child who is unable or unwilling to take an oral sedative.
- *An IV catheter* may be inserted in older children and adolescents while they are awake. A nurse can first numb the child's hand with a local anesthetic (EMLA cream) so that he will not feel pain when the catheter is inserted.
- *A mask induction* may be appropriate for some children. The child inhales an anesthetic gas through a mask. Often this form of induction is not used for children with brain tumors because they may have other problems (such as intracranial hypertension with vomiting) that would not make this a good choice.

Hospitals have different protocols for delivering anesthesia, and most work very well. No one wants this experience to be unpleasant for your child. In most cases, the choice depends on the individual patient and the specific situation. During the pre-operative visit, you may wish to ask your child's anesthesiologist why a particular method will be used.

Often while a child is undergoing brain surgery a nurse liaison will convey information from the surgeon to the family in the waiting room. As soon as possible after your child's operation, the surgeon will give you a preliminary report of how things went.

After the operation, the child generally goes to the ICU for overnight observation. A very small percentage of patients (for instance, those whose tumors affect the brain stem) remain intubated with an endotracheal tube and are kept under anesthesia for a while to let them have a chance to heal and recover before they have to breathe fully on their own.

In most cases, the endotracheal tube is removed in the operating room after surgery has been completed and anesthesia has been discontinued. The health care team will check the child's neurological function and provide pain medication. Most major centers that treat children with brain tumors also have a pain team in place. Because children can't always articulate the pain they are experiencing, this team helps to recognize early, sometimes subtle signs and helps manage pain before the child is in a lot of discomfort. "In the immediate postoperative period following a brain tumor resection, we give the patient narcotics. There's no benefit in having a child uncomfortable and in pain. The child is usually relaxed and drowsy by the time he gets to the ICU," says Dr. Rockoff. "Sleepy is okay."

Specialists in critical care medicine, called intensivists, will generally observe a child closely during the night following a craniotomy.

Recovery

The course of the child's recovery will depend on the type of procedure. If the child has had a stereotactic biopsy (see p. 141), (s)he may be up and about the same day. If (s)he has had a craniotomy (see p. 142), (s)he may require many days before she is feeling up to normal. Usually, after one night in the ICU, the child goes to a regular floor in the hospital.

The complications of pediatric tumor surgery are similar to those associated with adult surgery. For children with tumors around the cerebellum, swallowing can be a problem. If the child's gag reflex is affected, he or she will not be able to eat and may need to have a nasogastric tube or even a temporary gastrostomy, a surgical opening into the stomach. Rarely, children with surgery in the cerebellum may have a syndrome in which they have difficulty speaking.

After a child has surgery to remove a brain tumor, a family's overwhelming concern is often, "What was it? Is it treatable? What can be done about it?" Naturally, families are eager to hear the answers to those questions as quickly as possible. However, it can often take a week or longer to get results back from the pathology department. It is more important for the pathologist to be correct than fast, because any therapy that's based on the wrong diagnosis won't be right.

Depending on the location of the tumor and how the child is doing after surgery, she may stay in the hospital from two days to two weeks or more to recover. By the time the health care team has the answer back from the neuropathologist (often in 3 to 7 days), the child often is up and about and in many cases has already gone home. Not to know what the mass was can be tough for families. In some cases, the family will have to come back to the hospital to discuss the results with the team after the child has been discharged.

Diagnosis

At our hospital, once we have the results back from pathology, the neurosurgeon, pathologist, oncologists, and radiation specialists all sit together and look at the radiological films from both before and after the operation. We determine what the tumor was, where it was, and if there is any tumor left after surgery. As a group, we work out a treatment plan that we all agree to and then we meet with the family to discuss the details of how we will coordinate care to treat the child.

If some of the tumor still remains, it is best to be as direct and clear as possible when talking with the child. For instance, you might say, "The doctor was able to take out some of the tumor, but there is some that he couldn't reach," or "The doctor took out the whole tumor, but there is a chance that it may come back. If it starts to grow again, there are things that we can do to take care of it." Children tend to ask more questions as time goes on. If you don't have the answer, tell your child that you will talk with an oncologist to get the information that she needs. The important thing is that she will know that her questions will be answered.

Other Treatments

Just as with brain tumors in adults, the array of treatment options, beyond emergency surgery to remove the tumor, can be confusing and over-whelming. In this section, I will tell you about the use of chemotherapy, radiation, and other drug therapies for children. As you explore different forms of treatment, you may wish to contact the Pediatric Brain Tumor Consortium (PBTC), which is made up of several individuals from ten leading brain tumor centers for children around the country. This group is devoted to finding new treatments for children with brain tumors. Their Web address is www.pbtc.org. Another important group is the Children's Oncology Group (COG, at www.curesearch.org), which runs clinical trials for children with brain tumors.

Radiation

As I explained in chapter 12, radiation therapy has evolved considerably in recent times. Our imaging and neurosurgical techniques have allowed us to radiate or remove just the tumor with less damage to other parts of the brain. For survivors of brain tumors, the quality of life after treatment is much better than it used to be.

Because radiation of the whole brain and/or spine can interfere with many functions related to a child's growth, we used to be strict about giving radiation to young children. Now, for certain small tumors that are highly curable with radiation, we do give highly focused radiation therapy, but usually only for tumors in the bottom portion of the brain (the posterior fossa), not those in the top part of the brain (the supratentorial area). We can give little doses just to the site of the tumor and nowhere else.

Months after radiation therapy, if the child's pituitary gland (the gland that secretes several key hormones) was in the radiation field, levels of growth hormone, cortisol, or thyroid-stimulating hormone may change. The risk for hormone deficiencies will depend very much on the amount of radiation the child received and the targeting of the radiation.

At our center, an endocrinologist sees all children who have had radiation treatment. Blood tests that the endocrinologist may order include:

- IGF-1 and IGF-BP-3 to screen for growth hormone deficiency
- Thyroid function tests to rule out hypothyroidism
- LH, FSH, and either testosterone (male) or estradiol (female)—to check hypothalamic-pituitary-gonadal function
- Morning cortisol level or DHEA-sulfate level to check hypothalamic-pituitary-gonadal axis function.

The good news is that all of these deficiencies can be treated: hypothyroidism by hormone replacement therapy with a drug called levothyroxine; growth hormone deficiency by recombinant human growth hormone; hypogonadism by estrogen and progesterone; and adrenal insufficiency by cortisone. Laurie Cohen, a pediatric neuro-endocrinologist at Children's Hospital in Boston, notes that some parents are concerned that growth hormone may cause the child's tumor to recur, but to date there is no evidence that this is a risk. She also emphasizes that after radiation therapy, an endocrinologist should continue to monitor the child's hormone levels periodically for the rest of his or her life.

Chemotherapy

We sometimes give chemotherapy to children under age three until they can receive radiation therapy more safely. We try to cure infants without radiation. For children with low-grade gliomas, we also use chemotherapy and try to delay radiation therapy to age ten. Scott Pomeroy, M.D., director of neurological neuro-oncology at Children's Hospital in Boston, says, "At first the goal was age seven, and now it's greater than age ten. Some people are wondering whether we can actually replace radiation with chemotherapy."

As I mentioned in chapter 13, just as radiation therapy used to affect the whole brain (or a large part of it), we used to give chemotherapy that affected any dividing cell in the entire body. Now we're trying to develop chemotherapeutic agents that are less toxic and more directed just to the brain tumor. These therapies have the potential to increase cure rates of pediatric brain tumors.

Because chemotherapy drugs are designed and approved by the FDA for adults (not children), almost all of the drugs we give to children are used on an "off-label" basis. The primary chemotherapy drugs that we give to children with brain tumors include:

- vincristine
- the platinum drugs (carboplatin or cis-platin)
- cyclophosphamide or lomustine (CCNU)
- etoposide (VP-16)
- temozolomide (Temodar), which is still undergoing testing in pediatric brain tumors; therefore we lack the long-term data to know how well this drug really works in children compared to adults.

A variety of other chemotherapy drugs are used less commonly for pediatric brain tumors than for other pediatric tumors; these drugs include adriamycin, actinomycin, and irinotecan. In addition, some drugs are injected into the spinal fluid to help reduce the need for craniospinal radiation therapy in children.

Novel Drug Therapies

In general, we don't give experimental therapies to children unless other treatments are not working. Although it depends on the tumor and the situation, usually these therapies are reserved for those whose tumors are either highly malignant or those for whom other options have been exhausted. That said, we are beginning to try some biologic therapies (which are becoming less experimental) at the very outset of treatment. For instance, for babies in whom high doses of radiation could cause severe neurological damage, we are injecting drugs into the cerebrospinal fluid (CSF) so that they go all around the brain and spine.

Palliative Care in Children

There is a time in the course of some brain tumors when nothing more can be done. A study published in the *New England Journal of Medicine* in February 2000 revealed that often parents' and medical caregivers' perceptions of care diverge dramatically at the end of a child's life. Whereas parents may be most concerned with the child's pain relief, doctors may continue to hold out the hope of a cure. No one wants to "give up" on a child.

If treatment is not working and your child has already suffered because of a brain tumor, the health care team may recommend that aggressive therapy be stopped. Some hospitals have programs that offer end-of-life care to help you provide the best experiences possible for your child. These programs may include a variety of caregivers, including social workers, pain (palliative care) consultants, psychologists, patient care coordinators, nurses, and chaplains. Counselors in these programs can provide emotional support as well as pain and symptom management. They can help the family maintain a comfortable everyday routine or plan a family vacation or a special experience that would be meaningful.

What can you say to a child who asks, "Am I dying?" Psychologist Gerald Koocher says that if he is not dying, you can reassure him. If he is, you can say there is no cure, but you will help him fight as long as possible and give him the best quality of life possible. People are often afraid that a person will become despondent and fall apart if he hears this bad news. "Human beings rarely do that," Koocher says. "They may be sad and cry, but they're going to cope. The important thing is a sense of support. People don't want to feel abandoned. They want to know if they're uncomfortable, there will be pain relief and they will be with someone. They need to be able to say, 'I'm scared, I'll miss you.'"

One way to approach this subject with a child is to ask, "Do you ever worry about dying?" If he says "no," you might say, "I'm glad you aren't, but if you are you can talk with me about it." If he says "yes," ask what he is thinking—and address those thoughts. Above all, keep talking. Children know when adults are changing the subject. Koocher recalls a conversation he had with a child who was upset about being in the hospital. His parents were afraid to tell him that his tumor was not responding to radiation and they didn't know what to say to him if he asked about death. The child had seen a story on TV about a girl who had died of a brain tumor, and he was eager to get out of the hospital because he thought if he stayed there he would certainly die—and he was afraid of being alone.

Koocher met with the family to talk about their religious beliefs and to forge these into a meaningful response the whole family could understand. Together they told the child that they had done everything they could do to fight the tumor, but that the treatment was not working. They explained that he would die, but that he was going to be with God. Dying wasn't going to hurt. If he had a headache, they could give him something that would help. They assured him that they were not going to leave him alone.

Like adults, children who are living with a brain tumor can be treated with a variety of therapies, including surgery, radiation, chemotherapy, and other drug therapies. In the next chapter, I will describe other supportive measures that can provide strength and comfort; these include support groups, counseling, and integrative therapies such as acupuncture and massage.

PART FIVE

---◾---

Recovery

After the diagnosis, the best-case scenario for a brain tumor patient is to make it through treatment successfully and resume life as a healthy person. Certainly, the odyssey of surgery, chemotherapy, radiation, and other treatments may leave their mark, either in physical or emotional scars, or both. Often my patients talk with me about the tension between wanting to go back to their normal lives and the realization that they've been changed significantly because of their brain tumor. I try to encourage them to get back to as normal a life as they can.

For about 40 percent of the patients I see, the brain tumor episode is simply a bump in their road and they can return to their full, active lives. They may have had a meningioma, pituitary adenoma, vestibular schwannoma, colloid cyst, pediatric pilocytic astrocytoma, or some other tumor that can have long-term remission. For them, wellness means trying to forget that they lived for a period of time with a health problem that could have irreparably harmed them.

About 20 percent of patients can go back to a relatively normal life, but they face the possibility of lingering effects from their tumor. They may worry about having a seizure or they may have some visual loss or a problem with their pituitary gland that they will have to regulate with medicine. This group includes some patients with the same tumors I just described and some patients with low-grade gliomas, childhood medulloblastomas, or choroid plexus papillomas.

The third group of patients are the true combatants—they fight a daily battle with their brain tumor and the deficits caused both by the tumor and by the treatment. These patients include adults or children with malignant gliomas; adults with metastatic brain tumors or with lymphomas; and children with malignant ependymomas and other tumors.

In this final part of the book, I will focus on how to recover a sense of wholeness after learning that you have a brain tumor and how to reenter the world after going through treatment. Last, I will highlight some of the many reasons why you can be hopeful as you work your way through the process of recovery.

18

—■—

Working Toward Wellness

I've learned the art of knowing how to pull what I need from different resources.

—Brain tumor survivor

For many patients, recovery begins at the moment of diagnosis, because once we have determined the cause of their headaches and other symptoms, we can begin to treat the tumor and assist them in getting back to their lives. Recovery does not always mean that a person will be able to move forward without symptoms, however. Often it involves a period of adjustment to either subtle or profound changes. In this chapter, people who live with inoperable brain tumors and people who have experienced surgery and other treatments for brain tumors will share their thoughts on what you and your family can expect as you begin to work your way toward "the new normal." Here you will also find advice on how nutritional, physical, and speech therapy; counseling and support groups; and integrative therapies (such as acupuncture and massage) can help you gradually regain your bearings in your personal and professional life.

Recovery from Surgery

I want to feel sharp again. I have trouble staying with conversations and my contributions are off the mark. I was never a know-it-all. I'd like to recover the confidence to say I don't know without

feeling stupid. I say it, but before the surgery I used to say it and still feel smart.
> —Suzy Becker, *I Had Brain Surgery, What's Your Excuse?*

Your tumor may respond to surgery and other treatment in one of three ways:

1. Partial response (or partial remission)—the tumor has shrunk a little bit or stopped growing.
2. Full response—the tumor is completely gone.
3. Remission—the symptoms or the tumor have disappeared (but are expected to return).

Even in cases where tumors have a full response, that is, are completely eradicated, a patient may still emerge from treatment with both physical and mental challenges. In terms of coping mentally, patients often find it difficult to tolerate a regimen of watching and waiting after a flurry of active treatment. If you find yourself in this situation, you will continue to have regular MRI scans to see if a new tumor has formed or the old one has grown. At times you may feel as though you are waiting for "the other shoe to drop"—for what you feel is the inevitable return of your tumor. Some of the strategies I shared with you in chapter 10 may be helpful if you feel like you are living MRI to MRI.

I've covered the possible side effects of treatment in previous chapters, and the after-effects are similar, ranging from general weakness to compromised function based on the location—or former location—of the tumor.

Strengthening Your Body

Many types of specialists can help you alleviate the physical consequences of brain tumor care:

- **Nutritionist:** Most hospitals have a nutritionist on staff who can suggest changes to make to your diet to promote optimal healing.
- **Speech and swallowing therapist:** A speech and language therapist (a speech-language pathologist) helps individuals not only regain their ability to communicate but overcome swallowing problems that may follow surgery or radiation therapy.

- **Occupational therapist (OT):** A professional who is trained to help people resume the activities of daily living: cooking, dressing, etc., as well as regain job skills. He or she will work with your strengths to help you compensate for any weaknesses in these areas.
- **Physiotherapist (PT):** A specialist trained to assess and improve a person's muscle strength, ability to walk, and other physical problems.
- **Physiatrist:** A medical doctor who specializes in rehabilitative medicine and can assess your physical strength and plan resources, such as physical therapy, which you might need.
- **Urologist:** This doctor specializes in kidney and bladder problems and can help with problems of incontinence or urinary tract infections.
- **Neuro-ophthalmologist:** If your tumor is interfering with your vision, you may wish to see an eye doctor who has expertise in both the eyes and the brain. He or she may be able to provide prisms for double vision or special lenses for visual field problems and may also refer you to a low-vision clinic.

These specialists can all help in making your recovery as effective as possible. Lisa Doherty, an oncology nurse practitioner at our hospital, recommends that you stay as active as you can and, no matter what type of extra therapy you do, always follow the recommended exercises to gain strength and get the benefits you want. None of these regimens will help much if you do not follow through with the prescribed maintenance exercises between your appointments.

Each patient's experience of recuperation is a little different. The length of time to get back to normal, and the effort required to do so, will depend on your age, the type of tumor you had (or have) and its location, how extensive your surgery was, and what your health was like before you discovered you had a brain tumor.

Strengthening Your Mind

In addition to physical therapy, you may need support because of memory loss, difficulty with attention, depression, and other emotional and psychological problems. Malcolm Rogers, a psychiatrist who works with our brain tumor group, says, "Depending on the precise location of the tumor, deficits may be more specific—such as the loss of ability for calculation or differentiation of right from left—or more subtle and generalized. They might simply involve a change in the speed of processing information or an alteration in judgment and insight. The deficits may be temporary or more permanent, depending on whether the cause is temporary swelling or permanent nerve damage in a particular part of the brain."

Many people who are recovering from a brain tumor also struggle with their identity. Anything that affects your brain can be threatening to who you are. One patient said, "I had part of my brain, part of my very mind removed." Another said, "This is the beginning of my new life and I'm dealing with all of these other things on top of the fear of its return, but I'm not the same person I was before. I can't work and can't do the same type of job."

Many of my patients—both children and adults—feel that they are fundamentally different than other people because they have or have had a brain tumor. Some have difficulty with a stigma that they perceive because of physical disfiguration from brain surgery or because of hair loss due to surgery, radiation, or chemotherapy. Others bear invisible psychological scars from their experience.

If you break your arm, everyone you encounter can see your injury and most will ask what happened and offer their sympathy. If you have a brain tumor, most likely you look exactly the same as you always have—and you have nothing to show for your troubles. Even so, the way you see yourself has changed, and people around you may notice changes in your behavior. You may be too tired to cook, or if you try, too weak to turn the spatula. Your children may wonder why you have suddenly grown "lazy." Dr. Rogers notes, "There is a tendency . . . arising from frustration, to think that someone is not trying hard enough or making certain mistakes on purpose, or even being selfish. A clarification that certain behavioral changes are neurologically based and beyond the patient's control can often be very helpful to families."

Specialists who can help you meet these challenges include:

- A **neuropsychologist** can diagnose your cognitive difficulties through either a brief mental status examination or more extensive neuropsychological tests. He or she most likely will want to meet both with you and with your family members to talk about these difficulties.

This type of specialist can also work with you in *cognitive retraining* to help one part of your brain assume the tasks of the part that has been injured.

- A **psychiatrist** can collaborate with others on the health care team to determine whether mental and behavioral symptoms are the result of the brain tumor, a psychological or stress reaction to the tumor, side effects from medication, or the effects of some other treatment such as radiation therapy. In addition to his or her role in diagnosing the problem, a psychiatrist can offer psychotherapy as well as drug therapy. Depending on the results of your neuropsychological tests, a psychiatrist may recommend medications such as antidepressants (for depression) or stimulants (to help you remain more alert and focused).

- A **behavioral neurologist** can assess and help to treat subtle changes in sensation, mood, and organizational ability. He or she can recommend appropriate therapies for these difficulties.

- A **licensed social worker** can offer "talk therapy" to help you express your fear and frustration and the effects of your experience on your relationships. This form of therapy can be a safe place to cope with your worry, which can consume the energy that you need to heal. Some social workers also facilitate support groups for people with brain tumors.

Most centers that treat patients with brain tumors have a team of mental health professionals on staff. If you live far away from or are otherwise unable to attend such a center, you might ask your primary care physician for a referral to a mental health professional in your community.

Support Groups

A support group can connect you with others who share your situation. These groups can help people feel less isolated (especially if they are not able to work); share information and hope; find mutual support; advocate for one another; and seek out information for one another. Sometimes people discover new ways to cope through these groups. People manage in different ways and some ways are healthier and more adaptive than others.

Types of Support Groups

There are groups for both adults and children with brain tumors, groups for family members, and groups for both. Family members can meet with one another to share strategies for handling all kinds of issues related to the diagnosis, from their loved one's memory loss to fear about the future.

If there is no brain tumor support group in your area, you may want to find a cancer wellness or support group. Often people with other types of tumors share the same concerns. Support groups for people who have experienced a head injury may also be helpful, especially if you are going through speech or physical therapy.

What Happens at a Support Group?

Groups are usually facilitated by a health or mental health professional (often a social worker) who guides the discussion and, if he or she cannot answer medical questions that arise, can recommend a person who can. There may be a guest speaker on topics such as nutrition and meditation, followed by a question-and-answer session and more informal discussion in small groups.

Ellen Golden, a social worker at our hospital who has run support groups for people with brain tumors, says that the subjects of discussion may include tumor types; treatments explored; new research or legislation; family dynamics; problems with working or not working; relationships with friends; and sometimes marital problems, separations, or in some cases, divorces that result from the difficulty of handling this major life change.

You might call the facilitator ahead of time to find out how the meetings are set up and where and when they take place. (At our hospital, they meet twice each month for an hour to two hours.) If you are uncomfortable about sharing your story with a group of strangers, you might want to send a friend to the first meeting in your place to see how it works. You may also take a friend or family member with you. You can share as much or as little information about your own situation as you wish.

Golden notes that, in her experience, "the group as a whole was very respectful of newcomers. We would open with a statement that people are

coming from different backgrounds and experiences. We asked partici-
pants to acknowledge that people can be in a difficult place, but everyone
should try to stay hopeful. People would usually come with a purpose or
question: 'This was my experience, what was yours?' We tried to find a balance to meet everyone's needs."

Befriending a Fellow Combatant

Some programs will match patients with the same diagnosis so that they
can support each other over the telephone. Some people don't like support
groups, but they like talking one-on-one. When asked which resources
have helped him the most, one patient said, "I befriended a fellow combatant." This college student, who was diagnosed with an astrocytoma at age
eighteen, befriended an eleven-year-old girl he met during treatment.
They still e-mail each other. He believes that this "buddy system" has
helped them both.

Lisa Doherty adds a word of caution about these relationships: When
two people are doing well, these types of connections can be encouraging.
But when one is doing well and the other is doing poorly, both parties may
experience depression and guilt. She advises patients to keep a social
worker or other professional counselor in the loop of their relationship.
You may wish to contact the American Brain Tumor Association for help
in finding a support group near you (800-886-2282).

Writing It Down

People sometimes establish e-mail or pen pal exchanges with acquain-
tances who they have met in support groups. The American Brain Tumor
Society (www.abts.org) also sponsors a "connections" pen pal program.

Both old-fashioned and online diaries can also be a good way to
express fears and frustrations that stem from the brain tumor experience.
The BBC reporter Ivan Noble found his online blog therapeutic:

> That personal style of journalism was never something I was particu-
> larly attracted to or interested in reading myself. But when I was diag-
> nosed back in 2002 I had a strong urge to fight back against what felt
> like the powerlessness of the situation. I really wanted to try to make
> something good out of bad.
>
> I was not sure if what I wrote would be any good and I was not
> sure if anyone would read it, but I wanted to try.

I know now that people have found the diary useful, and it meant a lot to me in particular to know that there were people in a similar situation to me or caring for such people who got something out of it. The regular feedback from dozens and dozens of people every time I have written has been wonderful, especially in real times of crisis. I know that it has kept me going much longer than I would have without it and I am grateful.

What I wanted to do with this column was try to prove that it was possible to survive and beat cancer and not to be crushed by it. Even though I have to take my leave now, I feel like I managed it.

Complementary and Alternative Therapies

Even as you pursue conventional therapeutic options (such as surgery, radiation, and chemotherapy), you may wonder if there is anything else you can do to fight your tumor and feel stronger. By now your health care team will have talked with you about the importance of good nutrition and physical activity. Some people also pursue complementary and/or alternative therapies to control the seizures, headaches, pain, anxiety, and fatigue that commonly accompany brain tumors.

I tell my patients that while they are receiving conventional treatment for a brain tumor, I don't mind if they also practice meditation, walk the labyrinth, try acupuncture, and explore other therapies as long as they tell me ahead of time so that we can ensure that these methods do not interfere with their treatment.

Generally, other than a daily vitamin, we don't recommend alternative medicines (drugs that have not been approved by the U.S. Food and Drug Administration) because some have never been tested and there has been little proven effectiveness from those that have been tested. (The FDA considers some herbs and supplements to be food—not medicine—so they are not tested as drugs.) We also don't know all of their potential side effects and interactions with the traditional medicinal therapies. In some cases these substances can reduce the effectiveness of other therapies. Some can promise miraculous results for a high fee; if it is going to cost a lot of money and there is no proven benefit, I discourage my patients from pursuing these remedies.

You may have heard various names for nonconventional types of therapies: alternative medicine, complementary medicine, and integrative therapies. What are the differences among them? According to the National Center for Complementary and Alternative Medicine (NCCAM), all of these forms of care fall outside the realm of conventional therapies that have been tested by scientific methods. *Alternative methods* are used in place of conventional ones. *Complementary methods* are used in addition to conventional ones. *Integrative therapies* combine, or integrate, conventional treatments with complementary ones for which there is "evidence-based" research that confirms their safety and usefulness.

Integrative therapies include diet and herbs; massage, acupuncture, and chiropractic care; naturopathy and homeopathy; mind-body therapies (yoga, meditation, and prayer); energy therapies (reiki, magnets, and qi gong); and music and art therapy.

According to David Rosenthal, M.D., medical director of the Leonard P. Zakim Center for Integrative Therapies at the Dana-Farber Cancer Institute in Boston, many of these therapies have one thing in common: they can reduce stress by triggering endorphins, the "feel-good" proteins in the brain that can help a person relax and produce a sense of well-being.

Diet and Herbs

A nutritionist at your hospital can advise you about your diet during conventional treatment for your brain tumor. In general, it is important to eat well at this time; restrictive diets can be harmful. The nutritionist can answer your questions about whether anti-oxidants and over-the-counter (OTC) botanicals will be helpful, not helpful, or even harmful. Some anti-oxidants interact poorly with chemotherapy drugs and radiation treatment. Again, a daily vitamin is usually fine, but don't take excessive amounts of vitamins, especially vitamins A and C.

Some people may feel a placebo effect from taking nutritional supplements, though we haven't found these to be curative. If you try these supplements, be sure to let your health care team know; they can check to ensure that these agents won't interfere with your chemotherapy regimen. Don't withhold this information out of concern that your doctors and nurses will disapprove of your decision to explore other therapeutic options. Your health care team shares your goals—they want you to get better and feel better.

Researchers have shown that some supplements (such as those that contain shark cartilage) can be toxic. Herbs such as garlic, gingko, and ginseng may cause bleeding. Ephedra may affect the heart. Kava can harm the liver. St. John's wort can reduce the effectiveness of chemotherapy drugs. The American Society of Clinical Oncology urges physicians and patients to remember: "These therapies should undergo rigorous scientific evaluation to measure their effectiveness and ensure that they do not interfere with conventional treatments."

Massage, Acupuncture, and Chiropractic Care

In addition to diet and herbs, complementary therapies include massage, acupuncture, and chiropractic care. In general, I believe these may help to alleviate pain and I encourage them as long as they are not too expensive for you.

Massage. More and more, massage therapists are working as life care specialists within hospitals. At our hospital, some people with brain tumors pursue massage therapy to help relieve neuropathy (nerve pain), headaches, insomnia, anxiety, depression, and nausea. Bambi Mathay, a massage therapist at the Dana-Farber Brigham and Women's Cancer Center, encourages patients to have their massages in the hospital (on an outpatient basis). She notes that in-hospital massage therapists "have access to your medical records and laboratory results, so we are up to date with what is going on."

Always check with your doctor before getting a massage. In some centers, the massage therapy team sends an "eligibility letter" to the person's doctor to ensure that massage would be safe at this time. Your doctor can confirm whether you:

- Are at risk for deep vein thrombosis (blood clots) and whether there are concerns that a massage may increase or decrease your blood clotting.
- Have a low blood platelet count (thrombocytopenia). If this count is lower than 10,000/ml, a massage could cause spontaneous bruising or bleeding.
- Have a low white blood cell count (neutropenia). If this count is low, your risk of infection is high.

Depending on where you are in your treatment, your massage therapist may give you a "light touch" massage with light to moderate pressure to help you relax, rather than a potentially injurious deep-tissue massage.

Acupuncture. Some people find that acupuncture helps ease their discomfort, nausea (from chemotherapy), fatigue, and anxiety. At our hospital, acupuncturists will work with patients who have brain tumors as long as their blood counts are high enough to fight off infection (over 25,000/ml platelets, over 500/ml absolute neutrophil count). We do not encourage this therapy for people who have abnormal heart rhythms or those who are planning to have or have recently had a stem cell transplant. You should not have acupuncture on parts of your body that have received radiation therapy because of potential further damage to already damaged skin.

If you pursue acupuncture, be sure to tell your health care team and see a licensed acupuncturist (Lac or LicAc); acupuncture with a licensed therapist is generally safe. Although the biomedical research community in the West did not formally embrace this type of care until the late 1990s, it is being used more and more with good results. One study of more than 34,000 patients who received acupuncture treatment found only 43 "minor adverse events" associated with this type of therapy. At the Dana-Farber Brigham and Women's Cancer Center in Boston, Dr. David Rosenthal notes that there have been no adverse events in more than 5,000 acupuncture treatments.

Many health insurance companies do not cover acupuncture.

Chiropractic care involves massage and manipulation of the body—especially the spine—to obtain relief from pain. It has a long history of antagonism with organized medicine because of a rather idiosyncratic view that human diseases start in the bones and skeleton. However, there is no question that chiropractic massage may help some patients.

Naturopathy and Homeopathy

Naturopathy and homeopathy have strong traditions in American medicine. Both are based on the concept that very small amounts of a medication might have a significant effect or that natural medicines may be as effective as pharmacological agents in effecting a change. Practitioners of these approaches come from a wide variety of backgrounds—from my point of view, it is only important that they be part of an integrative medicine program at a major institution and that the ingredients of their compounds have been reviewed to be sure there are no adverse interactions with other medications.

At our hospital, Susan DeCristofaro, R.N., M.S., O.C.N., teaches some of our patients with brain tumors about these approaches. She notes that naturopathy embraces a comprehensive program of lifestyle, diet, and herbs. Homeopathy involves the use of highly diluted minerals and animal and plant matter. She recommends that patients who pursue these treatment approaches see practitioners who have a medical license. An osteopathic doctor (D.O.) sometimes has training in these methods.

Mind-Body Therapies: Yoga, Meditation, and Prayer

> My prayer: I believe in friendship and loyalty. I believe in God's love. I believe in life.
> —A. J. Kirwan, diagnosed with an astrocytoma
> eleven years ago

Stress reduction, which can be achieved by yoga, meditation, and prayer, is an important part of any tumor recovery program. Imagery (imagining, for example, an island oasis where you are safe and untouched by pain) and visualization (for instance, concentrating on your good cells overpowering your bad ones) can also help a great deal.

Elana Rosenbaum, who has been teaching mindfulness, or insight meditation, techniques for more than twenty years, says that "mindfulness-based stress reduction" is a practical way to help people accept what is happening during difficult times. She notes, "Meditation brings attention to one's direct experience as it unfolds moment by moment without judgment. It enhances awareness and develops greater equanimity and peace of mind. If you can be present with it [the situation] rather than resist what is happening, you can make decisions that are more informed and less reactive."

Meditation is one way to directly work with fear. "Don't get lost in worries about the future or regrets about the past," Rosenbaum says, "because in the present moment there is some control." She found these techniques helpful when she was diagnosed with Hodgkin's lymphoma.

Meditation can be a wonderful tool that can help you stay calm during an MRI and radiation therapy. In sessions at our hospital, Rosenbaum teaches three types of meditation: mindfulness or "being present in the moment" meditation; body scan meditation, and loving-kindness meditation. The first, "being present in the moment," involves focusing on your breathing (or thoughts or sensations as they arise). Simply listening—which anyone can do at any time and any place—and breathing in and out, focusing on breathing and relaxing, can help to break up other thoughts and help you find a sense of calm and quiet.

Body scan meditation involves breathing and concentrating on the parts of the body—moving from the bottom of the foot up to the top of the head. This form of meditation can help in working through sensations that are difficult or painful—either eliminating them or learning to incorporate them into life.

Loving-kindness meditation includes three phrases: "May I be safe and protected," "May I be happy," and "May I experience health and a sense of well-being. May I live with ease." While Rosenbaum was recovering from her own stem-cell transplant, she wrote the following and referred to it often:

> I resolve to dwell in the present and not be captured by fear. I shall use my experience to remember the preciousness of life and the gifts I have received. I shall challenge myself to live wisely and make meaning of my experience, letting it transform me. I shall work to bring peace to others, so they, too, may be free. I am filled with gratitude to all who have helped me be alive and well. May I never forget the grace that has been bestowed upon me.
>
> It is not important what will be tomorrow. It is important to live today in harmony with myself and others and use the love I receive to give it out again. I shall work to maintain a balance, opening up to what is true, and acting accordingly. I shall not be ashamed of praise but value my efforts, appreciate my bravery, and celebrate my joy. May I be able to: enjoy, replenish, dance, and sing; make love; care fully for my body and the spirit, and help others do the same.
>
> May we all be well, and may I live with ease and happiness.

Energy Therapies: Reiki, Magnets, and Qi Gong

Reiki is a form of therapy that involves manipulations of energy fields within and around the body. DeCristofaro describes this energy as the "universal energy" that makes birds fly and seeds grow in the earth. Practitioners of reiki (called reiki masters) first evaluate the patient's needs and then "harness" this energy with the patient. While the person is lying quietly, the practitioner touches him or her to promote healing. This method, which may work by eliciting the relaxation response, can help to promote sleep and ease confusion and anxiety. In some states, reiki is taught in nursing schools.

Magnets, the placement of electromagnets on the body to ease pain and promote healing, and *qi* (energy) *gong* (skill) are similar concepts. These therapies do not appear to have any untoward effects.

Qi gong is a form of Japanese healing that is based on the concept of energy meridian points in the body. Our hospital offers classes in this type of low-impact exercise, which can be done while standing or sitting in a chair. People with physical disabilities can do this exercise with blocks and positioning equipment. During qi gong classes, patients concentrate on moving energy into parts of the body like the lungs, kidneys, and knees. Qi gong can help patients with brain tumors who may be experiencing trouble with balance and gait.

Music and Art Therapy

I think that music and art have the capacity to express emotions that are beyond words. I therefore strongly believe in using music and art to express ideas or approaches that are otherwise difficult. Again, making sure that therapists who offer these alternatives are part of an institutional approach and that they do not charge exorbitant fees are the only precautions I suggest. Insurance virtually never covers their cost.

More and more hospitals are offering creative arts programs for patients with brain tumors. Our hospital, for instance, offers instruction for patients who want to learn to play the piano, clarinet, guitar, or cello. Some take voice lessons. Musicians volunteer to work one-on-one with patients and patients perform in concerts on occasion.

At the Dana-Farber Cancer Institute, a theater workshop composed of patients, doctors, and hospital staff produced a play called *Adventures of Cell Zappers.* This year the group is going to produce *Wit,* a play about ovarian cancer. We also have a creative writing workshop and an artists' studio with a resident artist who oversees the program.

Seeking Joy

> I like nonsense, it wakes up the brain cells. Fantasy is a necessary ingredient in living, it's a way of looking at life through the wrong end of a telescope. Which is what I do, and that enables you to laugh at life's realities.
>
> —Dr. Theodore Geisel, a.k.a. Dr. Seuss

As you look into all of the resources that are available to you, remember to focus often on one of the oldest and most effective therapies available: laughter.

Several years ago, patients were giving our staff feedback about the serious atmosphere of the hospital. The response was a "humor initiative" called "Humor Us Healers." Both volunteers and some staff members now appear in clown costumes occasionally. They visit both pediatric and adult patients and sometimes appear at medical conferences to provide a little bit of entertainment.

My colleague David Rosenthal often wears a shirt that says, "Humor is the best medicine." Humor does help. One night one of my patients had just had it. He wanted to rip out his IV lines and leave the hospital. Someone called his favorite nurse, who appeared and helped him throw a "pity party." The whole episode ended with them both laughing hysterically.

In the book *I Had Brain Surgery, What's Your Excuse?* the artist and writer Suzy Becker discusses her recovery from brain surgery:

> I regained, in some ways found, an appreciation for a lot of things. Cartooning was a big one. I never realized how finding the humor in things, circumstances, gives me a feeling of power over them. . . . Just looking for humor—I'm lucky that's what I do.
>
> I like to think I got better at accepting help. I know I learned a lot about offering it. Maybe I'm a little less of a perfectionist.

A patient said, "It's not enough to be just alive." If you have a positive outlook and support from your family, friends, colleagues, and your health care team, you will do better. Lean on other people until you get your strength back. Above all, know that you can be the exception no matter what the disease. There is always hope.

19

■

Reasons for Hope

In the midst of winter, I found there was, within me, an invincible summer.

—Albert Camus, French philosopher

Hope begins in the dark, the stubborn hope that if you just show up and try to do the right thing, the dawn will come.

—Anne Lamott, *Bird by Bird: Some Instructions on Writing and Life*

It was like having a second chance.

—Beau Dyer, brain tumor survivor

It's challenging and it's been a blessing.

—Amy Masso, brain tumor combatant

We're here and we're spiritual beings having human experiences.

—A brain tumor patient of five years

I work better than before. I put more effort into everything that I do. Before I was happy with B's; now I want A's.

—Tim Barrett, survivor of a glioma for six years

I live a very magical life and I feel such gratitude.

—Woman who has fought an astrocytoma for eight years

It would be so lovely for us all to set cancer aside for three months and not even be able to comprehend the name. But that is not possible and wishing for miracles is a silly waste of time in precious days.

But I believe that cancer is losing. Cancer succumbs all the time both to the incremental improvements of science and the determination of those of us living and surviving the disease day by day.

Cancer will lose and people will win.

—Ivan Noble, BBC reporter

When I started working here five years ago, we had just a few options. Now we have many. There are medications with less side effects. More money is being spent on brain tumor research and we are learning about why some grow and some resist medications. Things are changing all the time.

—Lisa Doherty, neuro-oncology nurse practitioner

If you have a brain tumor or have a friend with a brain tumor, you may want desperately to know whether there is any hope. The answer is: yes.

There are many reasons for this. The tumor may be incidental and not need to be treated at all; the initial treatment may produce a cure or at least long-term remission; better and better treatments are being developed for malignant tumors; the outcome for you is completely unknown no matter what the statistics say; and more and more resources are available to help you in your journey even if you have a malignant tumor that is not responding to therapy.

Many people think a brain tumor is equivalent to a death sentence. Statistical research and my own patients' experiences show that this is far from the actual truth. Whatever stage you're in—whether you've just been diagnosed with a brain tumor, are undergoing treatment, or are looking forward to recovery—remember that there's always reason to hope.

- **Not all brain tumors require treatment.** In Parts Two and Three we learned that tumors come in all shapes, sizes, and behaviors and considered "watching and waiting" as a treatment plan for some tumors. At least 20 percent of the patients I see for the first time will not need immediate treatment for their tumor. Some of them have small benign tumors, some have cysts that will probably not grow, and some have abnormal MRI scans that may or may not represent a tumor. You can live a perfectly normal life with these conditions.

- **The tumor may be treatable.** Many of the patients I see with brain tumors have slow-growing, well-encapsulated tumors that can be dealt with successfully with observation, surgery, or focused radiation. In the chapters on tumor types, surgery, and radiation, we discussed many tumors that could be treated effectively with surgery. These include most meningiomas, vestibular schwannomas, pituitary adenomas, colloid cysts, epidermoids, lipomas, pineocytomas, choroid plexus papillomas, and pilocytic astrocytomas. These tumors need not affect your quality of life, your survival, or your brain function. As surgery gets more and more minimally invasive, we are able to remove these tumors with special surgical techniques— microsurgery, image-guided surgery, and intraoperative imaging.

There are also many tumors that can be controlled well with contemporary neurosurgical techniques even if they cannot be completely cured. These include low-grade gliomas, including oligodendrogliomas and astrocytomas; dysembryoplastic neuroepithelial tumors; craniopharyngiomas; neurocytomas; spinal cord gliomas; and ependymomas. For the majority of my patients, these tumors can be removed and followed for many years without having terrible effects on the patient or his or her family.

- **There are better and better treatments for primary malignant tumors.** About 50 percent of the tumors a neurosurgeon sees can be dealt with satisfactorily with surgery alone. That leaves about half that are difficult to treat; often these tumors are malignant. Among primary brain tumors, these include anaplastic oligodendrogliomas and astrocytomas, lymphomas, and glioblastomas. There have been great strides in managing all of these tumor types. We now have specific chemotherapies based on the molecular biology of the tumor. We have new chemotherapeutic strategies to fight lymphomas. For glioblastomas, we have targeted therapies and anti-angiogenic treatments as well as better, less invasive, more effective surgery.

- **There are better and better treatments for metastatic brain tumors.** A decade ago, a brain metastasis was thought to be untreatable and fatal. Today, using image-guided surgery, intraoperative imaging, and radiosurgery, we can very often deal with the metastasis extremely well. Symptoms can be relieved and survival rates can be improved.
- **The outcome for any person is not predicted by the statistics.** It is a fallacy of logic to take the concept that 95 percent of patients with glioblastoma die within five years and extrapolate to say that you have a 95 percent chance of being dead in five years if you have this diagnosis. Statistics are meant for large populations, not for individual people. You are either dead or alive—there is no ambiguity involved. No one has your particular set of genes, immune responses, and tumor cells. As doctors, we make some predictions, but we cannot anticipate what *your* body and immune system will do.
- **Even if you have a malignant brain tumor and are not responding to therapy, there are ever-increasing resources to help you and your family cope.** Everyone dies sometime. The issue is what kind of death it is—is it painful and lonely and bitter?—or is it a death surrounded by friends and family, happy in what you have done to try to defeat death, and at peace with yourself and your environment?

Two poems always stick in my mind about the approach to death, and I include them here. The first is by the poet Dylan Thomas, who was writing about admonishing his father as he was dying not to give up. This might be the theme of many of my patients who want to do everything possible to prolong their time on earth.

Do Not Go Gentle into That Good Night

Do not go gentle into that good night,
Old age should burn and rave at close of day;
Rage, rage against the dying of the light.

Though wise men at their end know dark is right,
Because their words had forked no lightning they
Do not go gentle into that good night.

Good men, the last wave by, crying how bright
Their frail deeds might have danced in a green bay.
Rage, rage against the dying of the light.

Wild men who caught and sang the sun in flight,
And learn, too late, they grieved it on its way,
Do not go gentle into that good night.

Grave men, near death, who see with blinding sight
Blind eyes could blaze like meteors and be gay,
Rage, rage against the dying of the light.

And you, my father, there on the sad height,
Curse, bless, me now with your fierce tears, I pray.
Do not go gentle into that good night.
Rage, rage against the dying of the light.

The second is a poem that is now four hundred years old, by the preacher John Donne, perhaps best known for his phrase "No man is an island." In this poem, he talks about how death is unjustifiably arrogant—it is not so special and it is not the end.

Death, Be Not Proud

Death, be not proud, though some have called thee
Mighty and dreadful, for thou are not so;
For those whom thou think'st thou dost overthrow
Die not, poor Death, nor yet canst thou kill me.
From rest and sleep, which but thy pictures be,
Much pleasure; then from thee much more must flow,
And soonest our best men with thee do go,
Rest of their bones, and soul's delivery.
Thou art slave to fate, chance, kings, and desperate men,
And dost with poison, war, and sickness dwell,
And poppy's charms can make us sleep as well
And better than thy stroke; why swell'st thou then?
One short sleep past, we wake eternally,
And death shall be no more; Death, thou shalt die.

The Promise of New Therapies

Translational Research

Ongoing research into the causes and treatment of brain tumors is making a difference. Perhaps the most promising steps in treating brain tumors better are to increase the molecular biological understanding of these tumors and then to begin to carry our knowledge from the clinic to the basic science laboratory and back again. This so-called translational research is critically important.

A number of new ideas will improve our ability to treat brain tumors. One is the concept that tumors might be treated by therapy "from the inside out." Instead of giving chemotherapy by intravenous infusion, for example, drugs can be delivered by techniques that involve direct delivery into the brain. These techniques include local infusion using a catheter placed into the tumor; slow-release polymers; and clusters of cells as molecular therapy agents.

There are also many new biological therapies—specific targets against EGF receptors, platelet-derived growth factor, and vascular endothelial growth factor; immune therapies; and drug combinations—which may be significant advances. These have been discussed in chapter 14.

Finally, new carrier agents for therapy—for example, stem cells for using molecular agents—may destroy these tumors. A growing cadre of scientists are looking for the Achilles' heel of malignant brain tumors to exploit it in the management of these tumors. Is it angiogenesis? Specific growth factors? The immune system?

There has never been a more optimistic time in the management of brain tumors, and as neurosurgeons and neuro-oncologists, we will do our best to bring these new developments to you.

Conclusion

If you or someone you love has a brain tumor, I hope that you have found the information in this book helpful. I have attempted to explain how patients who are living with a brain tumor can navigate their way through diagnostic tests and treatments and arrive at a changed, but good and meaningful life.

There is still a little more to this book—an appendix, which has further detailed information about topics we have discussed, suggestions for further reading, and resources. Beyond the book, however, there is you—the personality, abilities, talents, fears, and hopes that make you so special. I hope that you, your family, and your friends will be able to deal effectively with the problems associated with a brain tumor, and that you will emerge victorious in the fight against this vicious opponent.

APPENDIX

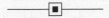

Statistics about Brain Tumors

Prevalence of Brain Tumors in the United States

- *Prevalence* is roughly the number of people who have a specific disease in the general population. The Central Brain Tumor Registry of the United States (CBTRUS) estimates that more than 359,000 adults were living with a diagnosis of primary brain and central nervous system tumors in 2000. More than 81,000 had malignant tumors, 267,000 had benign tumors, and 10,000 or more had tumors of uncertain behavior. (The reason there are so many more with benign tumors is that people with these tumors live a long time.) The prevalence rate for primary brain and central nervous system tumors was 29.5 tumors per 100,000 people (malignant); 97.5 tumors per 100,000 people (benign); and 3.8 tumors per 100,000 people (uncertain behavior): The prevalence rate for all primary brain and central nervous system tumors was estimated to be 130.8 tumors per 100,000 people.
- For pediatric tumors, according to CBTRUS, the prevalence rate for all pediatric (ages 0–19) primary brain and central nervous system tumors was estimated at 9.5 tumors per 100,000 people, with more than 26,000 children living with this diagnosis in the United States in 2000. The prevalence rate for pediatric primary malignant brain and central nervous system tumors was 7.9 tumors per 100,000 people, with more than 21,000 children living

with a diagnosis of primary malignant brain/central nervous system tumor in the United States in 2000.

Annual Incidence of Brain Tumors

The incidence of a disease is the number of new cases per year.

1. According to CBTRUS:
   - An estimated 43,800 new cases of primary brain and central nervous system tumors were expected to be diagnosed in the United States in 2005.
   - The incidence rate of all primary nonmalignant and malignant brain and central nervous system tumors is 14.8 tumor cases per 100,000 people. The rate is higher in females (15.1 per 100,000 person-years) than males (14.5 per 100,000 person-years).
   - This rate is 7.4 per 100,000 person-years for benign or borderline tumors and 7.4 per 100,000 person-years for malignant tumors.
2. According to the Surveillance, Epidemiology, and End Results (SEER) database:
   - The incidence of primary *malignant* brain and central nervous system tumors (excluding lymphomas, leukemias, tumors of pituitary and pineal glands, and olfactory tumors of the nasal cavity) is 6.4 tumor cases per 100,000 people. This rate is higher in males (7.6 tumors per 100,000 people) than females (5.3 tumors per 100,000 people).
3. According to the International Agency for Research on Cancer (IARC):
   - The worldwide incidence rate of primary malignant brain and central nervous system tumors, age-adjusted using the world standard population, is 3.7 tumors per 100,000 people in males and 2.6 tumors per 100,000 people in females. The incidence rates are higher in more developed countries (males: 5.8 tumors per 100,000 people; females: 4.1 tumors per 100,000 people) than in less developed countries (males: 3.0 tumors per 100,000 people; females: 2.1 tumors per 100,000 people). NOTE: these data include only malignant brain tumors.
4. Incidence of Pediatric Brain Tumors (ages 0–19):
   - The incidence rate of childhood primary non-malignant and malignant brain and central nervous system tumors is 4.3 cases per 100,000 person-years. The rate is higher in males (4.5 per 100,000 person-years) than females (4.0 per 100,000 person-years).
   - According to CBTRUS, an estimated 3,410 new cases of childhood primary nonmalignant and malignant brain and central nervous system tumors were expected to be diagnosed in the United States in 2005. Of these 3,410 new cases, an estimated 2,590 will be in children less than 15 years of age.

Lifetime Risk for Brain Tumors

- SEER: Males have a 0.65 percent lifetime risk of being diagnosed with a primary malignant brain/central nervous system tumor and 0.49 percent chance of dying from a brain/central nervous system tumor (excluding lymphomas, leukemias, tumors of pituitary and pineal glands, and olfactory tumors of the nasal cavity).
- SEER: Females have a 0.50 percent lifetime risk of being diagnosed with a primary malignant brain/central nervous system tumor and a 0.39 percent chance of dying from a brain/central nervous system tumor (excluding lymphomas, leukemias, tumors of pituitary and pineal glands, and olfactory tumors of the nasal cavity).

Survival Rates

- SEER: The five-year relative survival rate following diagnosis of a primary malignant brain and central nervous system tumor (including lymphomas and leukemias, tumors of the pituitary and pineal glands, and olfactory tumors of the nasal cavity) is 28.1 percent for males and 30.5 percent for females (1973–2002 data). However, these data are a combined figure that do not reflect the diversity of tumor types.

Adapted from SEER.cancer.gov and CBTRUS (2005) Statistical Report: Primary Brain Tumors in the United States, 1998–2002. Published by the Central Brain Tumor Registry of the United States.

Types of Brain Tumors

WHO Classification of Brain Tumors

Primary Brain Tumors

In the following table, the number in brackets describes the behavior of tumors:
   (0) benign tumors
   (1) low or uncertain malignant potential or borderline malignancy
   (2) in situ lesions
   (3) malignant tumors
These are based on the International Classification of Diseases for Oncology (ICDO) and Systematized Nomenclature Medicine (SNOMED).

Adapted from Paul Kleihues and Webster K. Cavenee. *World Health Organization Classification of Tumours: Pathology and Genetics: Tumours of the Nervous System.* Lyon, France: IARC Press, 2000.

Tumors of Neuroepithelial Tissue

ASTROCYTIC TUMORS
  Diffuse astrocytoma (3)
    Fibrillary astroctytoma (3)
    Protoplasmic astrocytoma (3)
    Gemistocytic astrocytoma (3)
  Anaplastic astrocytoma (3)
Glioblastoma (3)
    Giant cell glioblastoma (3)
    Gliosarcoma (3)
  Pilocytic astrocytoma (1)
  Pleomorphic xanthoastrocytoma
    (3)
  Subependymal giant cell
    astrocytoma (1)

OLIGODENDROGLIAL TUMORS
  Oligodendroglioma (3)
  Anaplastic oligodendroglioma (3)

MIXED GLIOMAS
  Oligoastrocytoma (3)
  Anaplastic oligoastrocytoma (3)

EPENDYMAL TUMORS
  Ependymoma (3)
    Cellular (3)
    Papillary (3)
    Clear cell (3)
    Tancytic (3)
  Anaplastic ependymoma (3)
  Myxopapillary ependymoma (1)
  Subependymoma (1)

CHOROID PLEXUS TUMORS
  Choroid plexus papilloma (0)
  Choroid plexus carcinoma (3)

GLIAL TUMORS OF UNCERTAIN
ORIGIN
  Astroblastoma (3)
  Gliomatosis cerebri (3)
  Choroid glioma of the third
    ventricle (1)

NEURONAL AND MIXED
NEURONAL-GLIAL TUMORS
  Gangliocytoma (0)
  Dysplastic gangliocytoma of
    cerebellum (0)
  Desmoplastic infantile astrocytoma
    (1)
  Dysembryoplastic neuroepithelial
    tumor (0)
  Ganglioglioma (1)
  Anaplastic ganglioglioma (3)
  Central neurocytoma (1)
  Cerebellar liponeurocytoma (1)
  Paraganglioma of the filum
    terminal (1)

NEUROBLASTIC TUMORS
  Olfactory neuroblastoma (3)
  Olfactory neuroepithelioma (3)
  Neuroblastoma of the adrenal gland
    and sympathetic nervous system
    (3)

PINEAL PARENCHYMAL TUMORS
  Pineocytoma (1)
  Pineoblastoma (3)
  Pineal parenchymal tumor of
    intermediate differentiation (3)

EMBRYONAL TUMORS
  Medulloepithelioma (3)
  Ependymoblastoma (3)
  Medulloblastoma (3)
    Desmoplastic medulloblastoma (3)
    Large cell medulloblastoma (3)
    Medullomyoblastoma (3)
    Melanotic medulloblastoma (3)
  Supratentorial primitive
    neuroectodermal tumor (PNET)
    (3)
    Neuroblastoma (3)
    Ganglioneuroblastoma (3)
  Atypical teratoid/rhabdoid tumor (3)

Tumors of Peripheral Nerves

SCHWANNOMA (NEURILEMMOMA, NEURINOMA)
  Cellular (0)
  Plexiform (0)
  Melanotic (0)

NEUROFIBROMA
  Plexiform (0)

PERINEURINOMA
  Intraneural perineurinoma (0)
  Soft tissue perineurinoma (0)

MALIGNANT PERIPHERAL NERVE SHEATH TUMOR (MPNST)
  Epithelioid (3)
  MPNST with divergent
    mesenchymal and/or epithelial
    differentiation (3)
  Melanotic (3)
  Melanotic psammomatous (3)

Tumors of the Meninges

MENINGIOMA
  Meningothelial (0)
  Fibrous (fibroblastic) (0)
  Transitional (0)
  Psammomatous (0)
  Angiomatous (0)
  Microcystic (0)
  Secretory (0)
  Lymphoplasmacyte-rich (0)
  Metaplastic (0)
  Clear cell (1)
  Chordoid (1)
  Atypical (1)
  Papillary (3)
  Rhabdoid (3)
  Anaplastic meningioma (3)

MESENCHYMAL NON-MENINGOTHELIAL TUMORS
  Lipoma (0)
  Angliolipoma (0)
  Hibernoma (0)
  Liposarcoma (3)
  Solitary fibrous tumor (0)
  Fibrosarcoma (3)
  Malignant fibrous histiocytoma
    (3)

  Leiomyoma (0)
  Leiomyosarcoma (3)
  Rhabdomyoma (0)
  Rhabdomyosarcoma (3)
  Chondroma (0)
  Chondrosarcoma (3)
  Osteoma (0)
  Osteosarcoma (3)
  Osteochondroma (0)
  Hemangioma (0)
  Epithelioid
    hemangioendothelioma (1)
  Hemangiopericytoma (1)
  Angiosarcoma (3)
  Kaposi sarcoma (3)

PRIMARY MELANOCYTIC LESIONS
  Diffuse melanocytosis (0)
  Melanocytoma (1)
  Malignant melanoma (3)
  Meningeal melanomatosis (3)

TUMORS OF UNCERTAIN HISTOGENESIS
  Hemangioblastoma (1)

Lymphomas and Hemopoietic Neoplasms

Malignant lymphomas (3)   Granulocytic sarcoma (3)
Plasmacytoma (3)

Germ-Cell Tumors

Germinoma (3)   Immature (3)
Embryonal carcinoma (3)   Teratoma with malignant
Yolk sac tumor (3)   transformation (3)
Choriocarcinoma (3)   Mixed germ-cell tumors (3)
Teratoma (1)
  Mature (0)

Tumors of the Sellar Region

Craniopharyngioma   Papillary
  Adamantinomatous   Granular cell tumor

Metastatic Tumors

All are malignant.

Making Decisions about Treatment

The Patient Self-Determination Act of 1990 (Public Law 101-508, Section 4206 and 4751) was enacted November 5, 1990, as part of the Omnibus Budget Reconciliation Act of 1990 (OBRA '90). "Patient self-determination" refers to the right of competent adults to make their own medical treatment decisions, and includes the right to complete advance directives, saying how and/or by whom decisions should be made in the future in the event the person becomes incapacitated and unable to make his or her own decisions. See www.palliativecare.org.

Living Will: www.livingwill.com has links to the forms in all fifty states.

Examples of a health-care proxy form and a living will from Brigham and Women's Hospital are reprinted here.

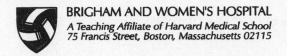

BRIGHAM AND WOMEN'S HOSPITAL
A Teaching Affiliate of Harvard Medical School
75 Francis Street, Boston, Massachusetts 02115

LIVING WILL DECLARATION

To My Family, Doctors, and All those Concerned with My Care:

I, _____, residing at _____
_____, make this statement to express my wishes regarding the withholding or withdrawal of life support should a time come when, as determined by my doctor, I am unable to participate in decisions regarding my health care.

Should a time come when there is no expectation of my recovery from physical or mental disability or disease, I direct that I be allowed to die with dignity, and that my doctor withhold or withdraw treatment that merely prolongs life and is unlikely to offer a cure or remission of the disease. I direct that my treatment be limited to measures that will keep me comfortable and relieve pain.

These directions are made after careful consideration and in accordance with my strong convictions and beliefs. I expect my family, doctor, and others concerned with my care to abide by my wishes and in doing so, to be free of any legal or moral liability.

Additional Instructions/comments: _____
_____
_____
_____

Signature: _____

Date: _____

HEALTH CARE PROXY

I, _____, residing at _____,
appoint _____, residing at _____,
telephone _____, as my health care agent with the authority to make
all health care decisions on my behalf. This authority becomes effective if my
attending physician determines in writing that I lack the capacity to make or
communicate health care decisions myself. My health care agent shall have the
same authority as I would to make these decisions. EXCEPT (LIST THE LIMITA-
TIONS IF ANY, YOU WISH TO PLACE ON THIS AUTHORITY):

_____

_____

I direct my health care agent to make decisions based on his/her assessment of my
personal wishes, including those expressed in the living will declaration I have
signed. Should my wishes be unknown, my agent shall make decisions based on
his/her assessment of my best interests. Photocopies of this proxy form shall
have the same force and effect as the original. If the person I have named is
unavailable, unwilling or not competent to serve, I designate the following person
as my alternate:

NAME: _____ ADDRESS: _____
_____ TELEPHONE: _____

Note: Generally, you may not choose as your health care agent an employee or mem-
ber of the medical staff of Brigham and Women's Hospital, unless you are related to
that person by blood, marriage or adoption.

_____   _____
Patient's Signature   Date

WITNESS STATEMENT
This form requires two witnesses 18 years of age or older:
We, the undersigned witnesses, each declare that we have witnessed the signing of
this document and that the person appears to be at least 18 years of age, of sound
mind and under no constraints or undue influence. Neither of us is named as the
health care agent or alternate.

Witness One: Witness Two:
Name (print) _____   Name (print) _____
Address: _____   Address: _____
Date: _____   Date: _____

_____   _____
(signed)   (signed)

REFERENCES AND FURTHER READING

---■---

What Is a Brain Tumor?

American Cancer Society. *Cancer Facts and Figures 2005.* Atlanta: American Cancer Society, 2005.

Ferlay, J., F. Bray, P. Pisani, and D. M. Parkin. *GLOBOCAN 2002: Cancer Incidence, Mortality and Prevalence Worldwide, Version 2.0, IARC Cancer Base no. 5.* (Lyon, France: IARC Press, 2004). Limited version available from: http:www.depdb.iarc.fr/globocan2002.htm.

Goldberg, Stephen. *Clinical Neuroanatomy Made Ridiculously Simple. Medmaster,* 2000.

Ries, L. A. G., M. P. Eisner, C. L. Kosary, et al., eds. *SEER Cancer Statistics Review, 1975–2002. (Bethesda, Md.: National Cancer Institute).* http:seer.cancer.gov/csr/1975_2002/. Based on November 2004 SEER data submission, posted to the SEER Web site 2005.

Stark-Vance, Virginia, and M. L. Dubay. *100 Questions and Answers about Brain Tumors.* Sudbury, Mass.: Jones and Bartlett, 2004.

Surveillance, Epidemiology and End Results (SEER) Program public use CD-ROM (1973–2002). National Cancer Institute, DCPC, Surveillance Program, Cancer Statistics Branch, issued April 2005, based on the November 2004 submission.

How Brain Tumors Are Diagnosed

Bromfield, Edward B. Seizures and Epilepsy Resulting from Brain Tumors. Watertown, Mass.: The Brain Tumor Society, 2005.

Castillo, Mauricio. *Neuroradiology Companion: Methods, Guidelines, and Imaging Fundamentals.* Philadelphia: Lippincott-Williams & Wilkins, 2005.

Gelb, Douglas. *Introduction to Clinical Neurology*. New York: Butterworth-Heinemann, 2005.

Types of Brain Tumors

Black, Peter, and Jay Loeffler. *Cancer of the Nervous System,* 2nd ed. Lippincott-Williams & Wilkins, 2005.

Burger, Peter, Stephen Vogel, and Bernd Scheithauer. "Surgical Pathology of the Nervous System and Its Coverings." London: Churchill Livingstone, 2002.

DeAngelis, Lisa. "Medical Progress: Brain Tumors." *New England Journal of Medicine* 344 (2001):114–23.

Kleihues, Paul, and Webster Cavanee. "World Health Organization Classification of Tumours: Pathology and Genetics: Tumours of the Nervous System." Lyon, France: IARC Press, 2000.

Levin, Victor. *Cancer in the Nervous System.* New York: Oxford University Press, 2002.

National Comprehensive Cancer Network. *The Complete Library of NCCN Clinical Practice Guidelines in Oncology* (2005).

How to Think about Treatment

Ali-Osman, F. *Brain Tumors.* Totowa, N.J.: Humana Press, 2005.

Zeltzer, P. *Brain Tumors: Leaving the Garden of Eden.* Encino, Calif.: Shilysca Press, 2004.

What a Brain Tumor Means for Me and My Family

Becker, S. *I Had Brain Surgery, What's Your Excuse?* New York: Workman, 2004.

Brain Tumor Society. *Color Me Hope: A Resource Guide.* Watertown, Mass. Available at www.tbts.org.

Holzemer, L. "Curveball." In press.

A Child with a Brain Tumor

Himelstein, B. P., J. M. Hilden, A. M. Boldt, D. Weissman. "Medical Progress: Pediatric Palliative Care." *New England Journal of Medicine* 350(2004):1752–62.

Hurwitz, C. A., J. Duncan, J. Wolfe. "Caring for the Child with Cancer at the Close of Life: "There Are People Who Make It, and I'm Hoping I'm One of Them." *Journal of the American Medical Association* 292(2004): 2141–49.

Kreicbergs, U., U. Valdimarsdottir, E. Onelov, et al. "Care-Related Distress: A Nationwide Study of Parents Who Lost Their Child to Cancer." *Journal of Clinical Oncology* 23(2005): 9162–71.

Mack, J. W., J. M. Hilden, J. Watterson, et al. "Parent and Physician Perspectives on Quality of Care at the End of Life in Children with Cancer." *Journal of Clinical Oncology* 23(2005): 9155–61.

Wolfe, L. "Should Parents Speak with a Dying Child about Impending Death?" *New England Journal of Medicine* 351(2004): 1251–53.

Watching and Waiting

National Comprehensive Cancer Network. NCCN Clinical Guidelines in Oncology 2005.

Surgery

Black, Peter, and Eugene Rossitch. *An Introduction to Neurosurgery.* New York: Oxford University Press, 1995.
Kaye, A., and P. Black. *Operative Neurosurgey.* New York: Churchill Livingstone, 1999.

Radiation

American Cancer Society. *Understanding Radiation Therapy: A Guide for Patients and Families.* Available at www.cancer.org.

Chemotherapy

DeAngelis, L. A., J. Y. Delattre, J. B. Posner. "Neurological Complications of Chemotherapy and Radiation Therapy." In M. J. Aminoff, ed. *Neurology and General Medicine,* 3rd ed. New York: Churchill Livingstone, 2001.
National Cancer Institute. "NCI Drug Dictionary." Available at http:cancer.gov/templates/drugdictionary.

Newer Therapies

Ernst, E. "The Risk-Benefit Profile of Commonly Used Herbal Therapies: Ginkgo, St. John's Wort, Ginseng, Echinacea, Saw Palmetto, and Kava." *Annals of Internal Medicine* 136 (January 1, 2002): 42–53.
MacPherson, H., et al. "The York Acupuncture Safety Study: Prospective Survey of 34,000 Treatments by Traditional Acupuncturists." *British Medical Journal* 323 (September 1, 2001): 486–87.
Sparreboom, A., et al. "Herbal Remedies in the United States: Potential Adverse Interactions with Anticancer Agents." *Journal of Clinical Oncology* 22 (June 15, 2004): 2489–2503.

Drugs for Swelling, Seizures and Other Problems

Samuels, M., S. Feske. *The Office Practice of Neurology.* London: Churchill Livingstone, 2003.

Choosing Supportive Care

Doyle, D., G. Hanks, N. Cherny, K. Calman. *Oxford Textbook of Palliative Medicine.* Oxford, Eng.: Oxford University Press, 2005.

Working toward Wellness

Levine, Margie. *Surviving Cancer.* New York: Broadway Books, 2001.

Reasons for Hope

Groopman, J. *The Anatomy of Hope.* New York: Random House, 2004.

RESOURCES

———■———

Note: The author and publisher do not specifically endorse the treatments or programs listed here, nor do they assume responsibility for their accuracy.

General Information about Brain Tumors

Central Brain Tumor Registry of the United States
244 East Ogden Ave., Suite 116
Hinsdale, IL 60521
630-655-4786
www.cbtrus.org

Surveillance, Epidemiology & End Results (SEER)
www.seer.cancer.gov

National Cancer Institute
www.NCI.nih.gov

Information on Specific Types of Brain Tumors

Acoustic Neuroma Association
P.O. Box 12402
Atlanta, GA 30355
404-237-8023
www.anausa.org

Acoustic Neuroma Association of Canada (ANA)
www.anac.ca

Meningioma Mommas
www.meningiomamommas.org

Pituitary Tumor Network Association
16350 Ventura Blvd., #231
Encino, CA 91436
805-499-9973
www.pituitary.com

Von Hippel-Lindau Family Alliance
171 Clinton Road
Brookline, MA 02445
800-767-4VHL
www.vhl.org

Centers that Treat Adults with Brain Tumors in the United States
(Based on data from the Society for Neuro-Oncology)

Alabama

University of Alabama
Brain Tumor Treatment and Research
    Program
Neurosurgery Dept: 205-934-7170
Neuro-Oncology Dept.: 205-934-7432
Birmingham, Alabama
www.braintumor.uab.edu

Arizona

Barrow Neurological Institute
St. Joseph's Hospital
Phoenix, Arizona
602-406-3181
www.thebni.com

California

Cedars-Sinai Medical Center
Maxine Dunitz Neurosurgical Institute
Los Angeles, California
310-423-7900
www.cedars-sinai.edu/nsi

City of Hope National Medical Center
Center for Neuro-Oncology
Duarte, California
626-256-4673 or 866-434-4673
www.cityofhope.org/cno/

Stanford University Medical Center
Neurosurgery Clinic
Stanford, California
650-736-1895
www.stanfordhospital.com/
    clinicsmedServices/clinics/
    neurosurgery/
    neurosurgeryClinic.html

University of California, Los Angeles
    (UCLA)
Brain Tumor Program, Dept. of
    Neurosurgery
Los Angeles, California
310-825-5111
www.neurosurgery.ucla.edu/programs/
    braintumor/braintumor_intro.html

University of California, San Francisco
Dept. of Neurological Surgery
San Francisco, California
415-353-7500
www.neurosurgery.medschool.ucsf.edu

USC/Norris Comprehensive Cancer
    Care Center and Hospital
Dept. of Neuro-Oncology
Los Angeles, California
800-872-2273
http://www.uscnorris.com/services/
    neuro_oncology/information.htm

Colorado

Colorado Neurological Institute
Englewood, Colorado
303-788-4600
www.thecni.org/braintumor

Connecticut

Yale University Brain Tumor Center
New Haven, Connecticut
203-785-2791
http:info.med.yale.edu/btumor/patients/
    firstvisit.html

Florida

Florida Hospital Neuroscience Institute
Brain Tumor Program
Orlando, Florida
407-303-1700

H. Lee Moffitt Cancer Center and
    Research Institute
Neuro-Oncology Program
Tampa, Florida
813-979-3980
www.moffitt.usf.edu

Shands at the University of Florida
Dept. of Neurosurgery
Gainesville, Florida
800-749-7424

Georgia

Winship Cancer Institute at Emory
    University
Neurosurgery Dept.
Atlanta, Georgia
888-WINSHIP or 404-778-3444
www.winshipcancerinstitute.org

Illinois

Chicago Institute of Neurosurgery and
    Neuroresearch (CINN)
Brain Tumor Program
Chicago, Illinois
800-411-CINN or 773-250-0400
www.cinn.org/ibsc/braintumor/
    braintumorhome.html

Evanston Hospital
Neuro-Oncology Program
Evanston, Illinois
847-570-1808
www.enh.org/healthandwellness/
    clinicalservices/neurosciences/
    index.asp

Loyola University Medical Center
Cardinal Bernadin Cancer Center—
    Neuro-Oncology Clinic
Maywood, Illinois
708-226-4357
http:www.luhs.org/svcline/cancer/
    service/c141.htm

Iowa

University of Iowa Hospitals
Holden Comprehensive Cancer Center
Brain Tumor Treatment Group
Iowa City, Iowa
800-777-8442

Maryland

Johns Hopkins University
Dept. of Neurology/Neurosurgery
Baltimore, Maryland
410-955-9441
www.neuro.jhmi.edu

UMM Greenebaum Cancer Center
Brain Tumor Center
Baltimore, Maryland
800-492-5538 or 410-328-7904
www.umm.edu/cancer

National Cancer Institute (NCI) and
    National Institutes of Health (NIH)
Brain Tumor Clinic
Bethesda, Maryland
Patient care coordinator: 301-402-6298
http://home.ccr.cancer.gov/nob

Massachusetts

Dana-Farber/Brigham and Women's
    Cancer Center
Brain Tumor Center
Boston, Massachusetts
617-732-6810
www.brighamandwomens.org/
    neurosurgery
www.dfci.harvard.edu

Dana-Farber/Children's Hospital Cancer
    Center, Boston
Brain Tumor Program
Boston, Massachusetts
617-355-6388
www.childrenshospital.org

Massachusetts General Hospital
Brain Tumor Center
Boston, Massachusetts
617-724-8770
http://brain.mgh.harvard.edu;
    neurosurgery.mgh.harvard.edu/
    nonc-hp.htm

Michigan

Henry Ford Hospital
Dept. of Neurosurgery
Detroit, Michigan
313-916-2241
www.henryfordhealth.org

Minnesota

University of Minnesota Hospital
Dept. of Neurosurgery
Minneapolis, Minnesota
www.neuro.umn.edu/

Mayo Clinic
Neurosurgery Dept.
Rochester, Minnesota
507-284-8008
www.mayoclinic.org/neurosurgery-rst/

New Jersey

New Jersey Neuroscience Institute at
    JFK Medical Center
Children's Neurological Center,
    Neuro-Oncology Dept., and Adult
    Neurosurgery
Edison, New Jersey
732-321-7000
www.njneuro.org

New York

Memorial Sloan-Kettering Cancer
    Center
New York, New York
212-639-7123
www.mskcc.org

Columbia University Medical Center
    Neurological Institute
New York, New York
212-305-6876

New York Weill Cornell Medical Center
New York, New York
212-746-8742

NYU Medical Center
Neurosurgery Dept.
New York, New York
212-263-6414
www.med.nyu.edu/neurosurgery

North Carolina

Duke University Medical System
Preston Robert Tisch Brain Tumor
   Center at Duke
Durham, North Carolina
919-684-5301
800-ASK-DUKE
www.cancer.duke.edu/btc/

Wake Forest University School of
   Medicine
Winston-Salem, North Carolina
Neurosurgery: 336-716-4081
Radiation Oncology: 336-716-4647
www.wfubmc.edu

Ohio

Cleveland Clinic Brain Tumor Institute
Cleveland, Ohio
800-223-2273 or 216-444-5670
www.clevelandclinic.org/neuroscience/
   treat/brain

Pennsylvania

Penn State Milton S. Hershey Medical
   Center
Neurosurgery
Hershey, Pennsylvania
800-243-1455
www.hmc.psu.edu/neurosurgery

University of Pittsburgh Cancer
   Institute
Brain Tumor Center
Pittsburgh, Pennsylvania
412-692-2600
www.neurosurgery.pitt.edu/braintumor

Thomas Jefferson University Medical
   Center
Dept. of Neurosurgery
Philadelphia, Pennsylvania
215-955-7000
www.jeffersonhospital.org/neurosurg

Tennessee

St. Jude Children's Research Hospital
Brain Tumor Program
Memphis, Tennessee
901-495-3604
www2.stjude.org/patient/cancers.htm

Vanderbilt University Medical Center
Dept. of Neurosurgery
Nashville, Tennessee
615-322-7417
www.mc.vanderbilt.edu/surgery/
   neurosrg

Texas

Dallas Children's Medical Center
Neuro-Oncology
Dallas, Texas
214-456-6139

University of Texas MD Anderson
   Cancer Center
Brain and Spinal Tumor Center
Houston, Texas
800-392-1611 or 713-792-6161
www.mdanderson.org/care_centers/
   brainspinal/

San Antonio Center for Neurological
   Sciences
University of Texas Health Science
   Center
San Antonio, Texas
210-567-5625
www.uthscsa.edu/neurosurgery

Utah

Huntsman Cancer Institute
Brain, Spine and Skull Base Tumor
    Service
Salt Lake City, Utah
801-585-0303 or 877-585-0303
www.hci.utah.edu/globalTop/
    contactHCI.jsp

University of Utah Health Sciences
    Center
Neuro-Oncology
Salt Lake City, Utah
801-585-0100
www.med.utah.edu/physref/
    department.cfm?D_ID=6

Virginia

University of Virginia Health System
Neuro-Oncology Center
Charlottesville, Virginia
434-982-4415

Washington

University of Washington Medical
    Center
Neurosurgery Clinic
Seattle, Washington
206-543-3572
www.uwmedicine.org

Virginia Mason Medical Center
Section of Neurology
Seattle, Washington
206-223-6881
www.virginiamason.org/dbNeurology/
    sec56973.htm

Wisconsin

University of Wisconsin-Madison
    Medical School
Neurosurgery Dept.
Madison, Wisconsin
608-263-1410
www.neurosurg.wisc.edu

Centers that Treat Adults with Brain Tumors in Canada

Ontario

Gerry and Nancy Pencer Brain Tumor
    Centre
Princess Margaret Hospital
Toronto, Ontario
416-946-2240
www.uhn.ca/programs/pencer

Hospital for Sick Children
Toronto, Ontario
416-813-8811
www.sickkids.ca/BTRC

Western Hospital
Toronto, Ontario
416-603-2581
www.unh.on.ca

Quebec

Montreal Neurological Institute and
    Hospital
Montreal, Quebec
Neurology: 514-398-6644
Neurosurgery: 514-398-1935
www.mni.mcgill.ca

National Consortia for Clinical Trials

North American Brain Tumor Coalition
    (NABTC)
www.nabraintumor.org

New Approaches to Brain Tumor
    Therapy (NABTT) Consortium
www.nabtt.org

Children's Oncology Group
www.childrensoncologygroup.org

Radiation Therapy Oncology Group
www.rtog.org

Financial Support for Medical Expenses

Cancer Care, Inc.
New York, New York
800-813-HOPE (4673); 212-302-2400
www.cancercare.org

Cancer Fund of America
Eastern Division: Knoxville, Tennessee
865-938-5281
Western Division: Mesa, Arizona
480-654-4715
www.cfoa.org

Drug Assistance Programs from
    Pharmaceutical Companies
Compiled by Supportive Cancer Care
Berkeley, California
510-649-8177
www.cancersupportivecare.com/
    drug_assistance.html

Kelly Heinz-Grundner Foundation
Wilmington, Delaware
www.khgfoundation.org

The Medicine Program
Doniphan, Missouri
573-996-7300
www.themedicineprogram.com/
    info.html

National Children's Cancer Society
St. Louis, Missouri
800-532-6459
www.children-cancer.com

Needy Meds
215-625-9609
www.needymeds.com

United Way
800-411-UWAY (8929)
www.unitedway.org

Lodging for Patients and Families:

American Cancer Society's Hope Lodge
www.cancer.org/frames.html

National Association for Hospital
  Hospitality Houses, Inc.
Asheville, North Carolina
800-542-9730
www.nahhh.org

Emergency/Medical Transportation

Aero-National
P.O. Box 538
Washington, PA 15301
800-245-9987

Air Ambulance America
9100 South Dadeland·Blvd., Suite 1104
Miami, FL 33156
301-695-2000

Aircare Alliance
Tulsa, Oklahoma
888-260-9707
918-745-0384
www.aircareall.org

Airlifeline
6133 Freeport Blvd.
Sacramento, CA 95822
800-446-1231
www.airlifeline.org

AirLineLift
1716 X Street
Sacramento, CA 95818
800-446-1231

Air Medical Alliance
3860 West Northwest Hwy,
  Suite 406
Dallas, TX 75220
800-687-4055

American Cancer Society
Note: Some local chapters reimburse
  patients for the costs of
  transportation to treatment.
800-ACS-2345
www.cancer.org

Angel Flight
3237 Douglas Loop South
Santa Monica, CA 90405
310-456-2035

Corporate Angel Network, Inc.
White Plains, New York
866-328-1313
914-328-1313
www.corpangelnetwork.org

DreamLine, Inc.
117 North Merrill Street
Park Ridge, IL 60068
847-910-3940
www.bobiverson.com/dreamline

Lifeline Pilots
www.lifelinepilots.org

Mercy Medical Airlift
800-296-1191
www.mercymedical.org

National Patient Air Transportation
  Hotline
Virginia Beach, Virginia
800-296-1217
www.npath.org

Family Support

National Association for Home Care
www.nahc.com

National Family Caregivers Association
10400 Connecticut Ave., Suite 500
Kensington, MD 20895-3944
800-896-3650
www.nfcacares.org

National Parent to Parent Support and
Information System, Inc.
P.O. Box 907
Blue Ridge, GA 30513
800-651-1151
www.NPPSIS@ellijay.com

Strength for Caring
www.strengthforcaring.com

Teens of Parent Survivors (TOPS)
www.braintrust.org

Well Spouse Foundation
30 East 40th St., Suite PH
New York, NY 10016
800-838-0879
www.wellspouse.org

Children and Brain Tumors

Adolescent Health Program
University of Minnesota
P.O. Box 721
420 Delaware St. SE
Minneapolis, MN 55455
612-626-2820

America's Baby Cancer Foundation
www.babycancer.com

Brain Tumor Foundation for Children,
Inc.
1835 Savoy Dr., Suite 316
Atlanta, GA 30341
770-458-5554
www.BTFCGAINC.org

Brave Kids
www.bravekids.org

Candlelighters Childhood Cancer
Family Alliance
www.candle.org

Candlelighters Childhood Cancer
Foundation (CCCF)
Kensington, Maryland
800-366-CCCF (2223)
www.candlelighters.org

Childhood Cancer Lifeline
www.childhoodcancerlifeline.org

Children's Brain Tumor Foundation
www.cbtf.org

Children's Cause
www.childrenscause.org

Children's Emergency Relief Foundation
and Children's Wish Foundation
International
www.childrenswish.org

Children's Hospice International
2202 Mt. Vernon Ave., Suite 3C
Alexandria, VA 22301
703-684-0330
www.chionline.org

Children's Tumor Foundation (formerly
  National Neurofibromatosis
  Foundation, Inc.)
www.ctf.org

Children's Wish Foundation
  International, Inc.
Atlanta, Georgia
800-323-WISH (9474)
770-393-WISH (9474)
www.childrenswish.org

Kids Cancer Network
P.O. Box 4545
Santa Barbara, CA 93140
805-693-1017
www.kidscancernetwork.org

Lighthouse SOS
www.lighthousesos.org

Make-A-Wish Foundation
Phoenix, Arizona
800-722-WISH (9474); 602-279-WISH
  (9474)
www.wish.org

Making Headway Foundation
115 King Street
Chappaqua, NY 10514-1615
914-238-8384
www.makingheadway.org

National Childhood Cancer Foundation
440 E. Huntington Dr., Suite 300
Arcadia, CA 91006
800-458-6223
www.nccf.org

National Children's Cancer Society
1015 Locust Bldg., Suite 600
St. Louis, MO 63101
800-532-6459
www.children-cancer.com

National Information Center for
  Children and Youth with Disabilities
P.O. Box 1492
Washington, DC 20013
800-695-0285
www.nichcy.org

Okizu Foundation Camps
16 Digital Dr., Suite 100
P.O. Box 6115
Novato, CA 94948-6115
415-382-9083
www.okizu.org

Pediatric Brain Tumor Foundation of
  the United States
315 Ridgefield Court
Asheville, NC 28806
800-253-6530
www.pbtfus.org

Pediatric Oncology Branch of the
  National Cancer Institute
www-dcs.nci.nih.gov/branches/pedonc/
  FAQ.html

Pediatric Oncology Group
www.pog.ufl.edu

Ronald McDonald Houses
1 Kroc Drive
Oak Brook, IL 60521
630-623-7048
www.rmhc.com

Starlight Foundation
www.starlight.org

St. Jude Children's Research Hospital
www2.stjude.org/patient/cancers.htm

Sunshine Foundation
Feasterville, Pennsylvania
215-396-4770
www.sunshinefoundation.org

Support Groups

Brain Tumor Society
www.tbts.org

Epilepsy Foundation
800-EFA-1000
www.epilepsyfoundation.org

Fertile Hope (for patients who are facing
cancer and fertility issues)
www.fertilehope.org

People Living with Cancer
www.plwc.org

Society for Neuro Oncology
www.sno.org

Taking the Fear Out of Cancer
www.takingthefearoutofcancer.com

Information about Radiation Therapy

Alopecia Areata Foundation
710 C St., Suite 11
San Rafael, CA 94901
415-456-4644
www.alopeciaareta.com

American College of Radiology
1891 Preston White Drive
Reston, VA 20191
703-648-8900
www.acr.org

The CyberKnife Society
www.cksociety.org

Elekta Instruments, Inc.
3155 Northwoods Parkway
Norcross, GA 30017
800-535-7355
www.elekta.com

International Radiosurgery Support
Association
P.O. Box 60950
Harrisburg, PA 17106-0950
717-671-1701
www.irsa.org

Look Good, Feel Better
Cosmetic, Toiletry, and Fragrance
Association
1101 17th St. NW, Suite 300
Washington, DC 20036
202-331-1770

Radiation Therapy Oncology Group
www.rtog.org

Soft Options
6345 Galletta Drive
Newark, CA 94560
510-787-8188

Tender Loving Care
American Cancer Society
1599 Clifton Rd. NE
Atlanta, GA 30329-4251
404-329-7776
www.cancer.org

Information on Chemotherapy

Alopecia Areata Foundation
710 C St., Suite 11
San Rafael, CA 94901
415-456-4644
www.alopeciaareta.com

Chemocare.com
www.chemocare.com

Chemotherapy Foundation
183 Madison Ave., Room 403
New York, NY 10016
212-213-9292

Look Good, Feel Better
Cosmetic, Toiletry, and Fragrance
　Association
1101 17th St. NW, Suite 300
Washington, DC 20036
202-331-1770

Medline
www.nlm.nih.gov/medlineplus/

Soft Options
6345 Galletta Drive
Newark, CA 94560
510-787-8188

Tender Loving Care
American Cancer Society
1599 Clifton Rd. NE
Atlanta, GA 30329-4251
404-329-7776
www.cancer.org

Newer Therapies and Clinical Trials

Cancer.gov/templates/drugdictionary

CenterWatch, Clinical Trials Listing
　Service
www.centerwatch.com

European Organisation for Research and
　Treatment of Cancer (EORTC)
www.eortc.be

Medicine Online
www.meds.com

Medline
www.nlm.nih.gov/medlineplus/

National Cancer Institute Clinical Trial
　Page
www.cancer.gov/clinical_trials/

National Center for Biotechnology
　Information
www.ncbi.nlm.nih.gov

PDQ List of Clinical Trials
www.cancer.gov/cancer_information

Pharmaceutical Research and
　Manufacturers of America
www.phrma.org

Musella Foundation: Clinical Trials and
　Noteworthy Treatments for Brain
　Tumors
www.virtualtrials.com

Information about Drugs

American Pain Foundation
www.painfoundation.org

Food and Drug Administration
www.fda.gov

Supportive Care

Hospice Alliance
www.hospice-alliance.com

Hospice Education Institute
www.hospiceworld.org

Hospice Foundation of America
2001 S. St. NW, Suite 300
Washington, DC 20009
202-638-5419
www.hospicefoundation.org

Hospice Hands
www.hospice-cares.com

Hospice Link
190 West Brook Rd., Suite 3-B
Essex, CT 06426
800-331-1620

National Association for Home Care
228 7th St. SE
Washington, DC 20003
202-547-7424
www.nahc.com

National Hospice and Palliative Care
  Organization
1901 N. Moore St., Suite 901
Arlington, VA 22209
800-658-8898
www.nhpco.org

Nursing Home Compare
www.medicare.gov/nhcompare/
  home.asp

Visiting Nurse Association of America
11 Beacon Street
Boston, MA 02108
888-866-8773
www.vnaa.org

Brain Tumors in Children: Clinical Trials

Children's Oncology Group
www.childrensoncologygroup.org

Centers that Treat Children with Brain Tumors

(Based on data from the Society for Neuro-Oncology)

Alabama

University of Alabama
1600 7th Ave. S.
Children's Hospital
Birmingham, AL 35294
205-939-9100

University of South Alabama
1504 Springhill Ave., Suite 5230
Mobile, AL 36604
251-405-5115
www.usouthal.edu

Arizona

Banner Children's Hospital
1450 South Dobson Rd., Suite 108
Mesa, AZ 85202
480-833-1123

Phoenix Children's Hospital
1919 E. Thomas Road
Phoenix, AZ 85016-7710
602-546-0920
www.phoenixchildrens.com

University of Arizona Health Sciences
    Center
1501 N. Campbell Avenue
P.O. Box 245073
Tucson, AZ 85724-5073
520-626-8278
www.crc.arizona.edu/research/
    cancer.htm

Arkansas

University of Arkansas
800 Marshall Street
Sturgis Bldg., 4th Floor
Little Rock, AR 72205
501-320-1494
www.archildrens.org/

California

Southern California Permanente
    Medical Group
9449 Imperial Hwy, Suite 342
Downey, CA 90242-2814
562-803-2479

City of Hope National Medical Center
1500 E. Duarte Road
Medical Office Bldg., 4th Floor
Duarte, CA 91010
626-256-4673
www.cityofhope.org

Loma Linda University Medical Center
11185 Mountain View Ave.,
    Suite 151
Loma Linda, CA 92354-2870
909-558-3374

Miller Children's Hospital/Harbor-
    UCLA
2801 Atlantic Avenue
Jonathan Jaques Cancer Center
Long Beach, CA 90801
562-933-8600
www.jjccc.com

Cedars-Sinai Medical Center
8700 Beverly Blvd.
Room AC1106, Lower Level Cancer Ctr.
Los Angeles, CA 90048-1865
910-423-4423
www.csmc.edu

Children's Hospital Los Angeles
4650 Sunset Blvd.
Los Angeles, CA 90027
323-669-2121
www.childrenshospitalla.org,
   www.purging.nant.org

UCLA School of Medicine
10833 Le Conte Ave., #A2-312
Division of Hem-Onc
Los Angeles, CA 90095-1752
310-825-6708

Children's Hospital Central California
9300 Valley Children's Place, FC13
Madera, CA 93638-8762
559-353-5480
www.childrenscentralcal.org/
   Specialties.asp?id=362

Children's Hospital Oakland
747 52nd Street
Oakland, CA 94609-1809
510-428-3689
www.childrenhospitaloakland.org

Children's Hospital of Orange County
455 S. Main Street
Orange, CA 92668
714-997-3000
www.choc.com

University of California, Irvine
101 The City Drive
Orange, CA 92868
714-456-6615

Stanford University Medical Center
725 Welch Road
Palo Alto, CA 94304
650-723-5535

Kaiser Permanente Medical Group, Inc.,
   Northern California
Pediatric Subspecialty
2025 Morse Ave., Station 1B
Sacramento, CA 95825
916-973-7342

Sutter Medical Center, Sacramento
5275 F St., Suite 2
Sacramento, CA 95819
916-733-1997
www.sutterhealth.org

University of California, Davis
UCD Medical Center Ticon II
2516 Stockton Blvd.
Sacramento, CA 95817
916-734-2782

Children's Hospital San Diego
3020 Children's Way, MC 5035
San Diego, CA 92123-4282
858-966-5811
www.chsd.org/

UCSF School of Medicine
505 Parnassus Avenue
San Francisco, CA 94143-0106
415-476-3831
www.pediatrics.medschool.ucsf.edu/
   hemonc/

Santa Barbara Cottage Children's
   Hospital
P.O. Box 689
Santa Barbara, CA 93105
805-569-8394
http:www.sbch.org

Colorado

The Children's Hospital
1056 19th Ave., #B115
Division of Pediatric Hem-Onc-BMT
Denver, CO 80218-1088
303-861-6740
www.thechildrenshospital.org

Presbyterian/St. Luke's Medical Center
 and CHOA
1800 Williams St., Suite 300
Denver, CO 80218
719-471-2462

Connecticut

Connecticut Children's Medical Center
282 Washington Street
Hartford, CT 06106
860-545-9630
www.ccmckids.org, www.ccmckids.org/
 services/hematology

Yale University School of Medicine
333 Cedar Street
P.O. Box 3333
New Haven, CT 06510-8064
203-785-4640

Delaware

Christiana Care Health Services/A.I.
 duPont Institute
1600 Rockland Road
Wilmington, DE 19899
302-651-5500
www.nemours.org/no/ncc/svcs/
 div545.html

District of Columbia

Children's National Medical Center
111 Michigan Ave. NW
Washington, DC 20010-2970
202-884-2800
www.dcchildrens.com

Georgetown University Medical Center
3800 Reservoir Rd. NW
Washington, DC 20007-2197
202-444-2224

Walter Reed Army Medical Center
 (USOC)
6900 Georgia Ave. NW
Ped/Hem/Onc Serv. Bldg. 2, Ward 52
Washington, DC 20307-5001
202-782-0421

Florida

Broward General Medical Center
1600 South Andrews Avenue
Ft. Lauderdale, FL 33316
954-355-4527
www.browardhealth.org

Children's Hospital of Southwest Florida
Lee Memorial Health System
9981 S. Healthpark Dr., Suite 156
Ft. Myers, FL 33908
239-432-3333

University of Florida
Shands Teaching Hospital
1600 SW Archer Road
Gainesville, FL 32610
352-392-5633

Joe DiMaggio Children's Hospital at
 Memorial
1150 N. 35th Ave., Suite 520
Hollywood, FL 33021
954-987-2000

Nemours Children's Clinic-Jacksonville
807 Children's Way
Jacksonville, FL 32207
904-390-3789
www.nemours.org/no/ncc/svcs/
    div545.html

Baptist Children's Hospital
8900 North Kendall Drive
Miami, FL 33176
786-593-1960
www.baptisthealth.net

Miami Children's Hospital
6125 SW 31st Street
Miami, FL 33155
305-662-8360
www.mch.com

University of Miami School of Medicine
P.O. Box 016960 (R-131)
Miami, FL 33101
305-585-5635

Florida Hospital Cancer Institute
2501 North Orange Ave., Suite 589
Orlando, FL 32804
407-303-2090
www.floridahospitalcancerinstitute.com
    /ChildrensProgram

Nemours Children's Clinic-Orlando
83 West Columbia Street
Orlando, FL 32806
407-650-7230
www.nemours.net

Sacred Heart Hospital
5153 N. 9th Avenue
Pensacola, FL 32504
850-505-4790

All Children's Hospital
880 Sixth St. S., Suite 290
St. Petersburg, FL 33701
727-767-7451
www.allkids.org, www.allkids.org/
    ACH_OncologyWeb/COG.htm

Tampa Children's Hospital
3001 W. Martin Luther King Jr. Blvd.
Tampa, FL 33607
813-870-4252
www.stjosephschildrens.com

St. Mary's Hospital
901 45th Street
West Palm Beach, FL 33407
561-840-6125

Georgia

Children's Healthcare of Atlanta, Emory
    University
2040 Ridgewood Dr. NE, Suite 100
Atlanta, GA 30322
404-727-4451
www.emory.edu/PEDS/HEMONC/

Medical College of Georgia Children's
    Medical Center
1120 15th Street
Augusta, GA 30912-3730
706-721-3626
www.mcg.edu

Backus Children's Hospital at MHUMC
4700 Waters Avenue
Savannah, GA 31404-6283
912-350-8194
www.memorialhealth.com

Hawaii

Cancer Research Center of Hawaii
1236 Lauhala St., #402
Honolulu, HI 95813
808-586-2979
www.crch.org

Tripler Army Medical Center (USOC)
MCHK-PE
1 Jarrett White Road
Tripler AMC, HI 96859-5000
808-433-6057

Idaho

Mountain States Tumor Institute
100 E. Idaho Street
Boise, ID 83712-6297
208-381-2711
www.slrmc.org

Illinois

Children's Memorial Medical Center at
    Chicago
2300 Children's Plaza
Box 30
Chicago, IL 60614
773-880-4562
www.childmmc.edu,
www.childrensmemorial.org

Rush-Presbyterian St. Luke's Medical
    Center
1753 W. Congress Pkwy
Chicago, IL 60612
312-942-5983

University of Chicago Comer Children's
    Hospital
5841 S. Maryland Ave., MC-4060
Chicago, IL 60637-1463
773-702-6808
www.ucch.org

University of Illinois
840 S. Wood Street
MC856, RM1245
Chicago, IL 60612-4325
312-996-6143
www.hospital.uic.edu

Loyola University Medical Center
Maguire Center, 3rd Fl.
2160 S. 1st Avenue
Maywood, IL 60153-5594
708-327-9135
www.luhs.org/rmch/

Advocate Hope Children's Hospital
4440 W. 95th St., Suite 4091H
Oak Lawn, IL 60453
708-346-4094
www.AdvocateHealthCare.com

Lutheran General Children's Medical
    Center
1775 W. Dempster St., 2nd Floor
Park Ridge, IL 60068-1174
847-723-5962

St. Jude Midwest Affiliate
530 NE Glen Oak
Peoria, IL 61637
309-624-4945

Southern Illinois University School of
    Medicine
801 N. Rutledge Street
P.O. Box 19230
Springfield, IL 62794-9230
217-785-2343

Indiana

Indiana University—Riley Children's
    Hospital
702 Barnhill Dr., #4340
Indianapolis, IN 46202-5225
317-274-8784

St. Vincent Children's Hospital
2001 W. 86th Street
Indianapolis, IN 46260
317-338-4673
www.stvincent.org

Iowa

Raymond Blank Children's Hospital
1212 Pleasant Street
Des Moines, IA 50309-1455
515-241-8912
www.blankchildrens.org

University of Iowa Hospitals and Clinics
200 Hawkins Drive
2528 JCP
Iowa City, IA 52242-1083
319-356-1905

Kansas

University of Kansas Medical Center
3901 Rainbow Blvd.
3032 Delp
Kansas City, KS 66160
913-588-6340
www.kumc.edu

Via Christi Regional Medical Center
929 N. St. Francis Street
Wichita, KS 67214
316-268-5691

Wesley Medical Center
929 N. St. Francis Street
St. Francis Campus, 7E (WCCOP)
Wichita, KS 67214
316-263-4311

Wichita Community Clinical Oncology
   Program
929 N. St. Francis Street
Wichita, KS 67214-3882
316-268-5784

Kentucky

A.B. Chandler Medical Center—
   University of Kentucky
Pediatric Hematology/Oncology
740 South Limestone St., J457
Lexington, KY 40506
859-323-5694
www.uky.edu

Kosair Children's Hospital
200 East Chestnut Street
Louisville, KY 40202-1822
502-852-8459

Louisiana

Children's of New Orleans/LSUMC
   CCOP
200 Henry Clay Avenue
New Orleans, LA 70118
504-896-9740

Ochsner Clinic
1516 Jefferson Highway
New Orleans, LA 70121
504- 842-5200

Tulane Univ./Tulane Univ. Hospital and
   Clinic
1430 Tulane Ave., SL-37
New Orleans, LA 70112
504-988-5412

Maine

Eastern Maine Medical Center
489 State Street
Bangor, ME 04401
207-945-7554

Maine Children's Cancer Program
100 Campus Dr., Unit 107
Scarborough, ME 04074-9308
207-885-7565

Maryland

Johns Hopkins Hospital
600 N. Wolfe Street
Baltimore, MD 21287-5001
410-955-7385

Sinai Hospital of Baltimore
2401 W. Belvedere Avenue
Baltimore, MD 21215
410-601-5864

University of Maryland at Baltimore
22 S. Greene Street, Suite N5E16
Baltimore, MD 21201
410-328-2808
www.umm.edu

National Cancer Institute—Pediatric
  Branch
10 Center Drive
Bethesda, Maryland
301-496-0085

Massachusetts

Dana-Farber Children's Cancer Center
44 Binney St., #SW-350
Boston, MA 02115
617-632-3791
www.dfci.harvard.edu

Massachusetts General Hospital
Yawkey 8B
Blake 2, Room 255
Boston, MA 02114
617-726-2000
cancer.mgh.harvard.edu/
  cancer_pedihemonc_home.htm

Baystate Medical Center
759 Chestnut Street
Springfield, MA 01199-0001
413-764-5316
www.baystatehealth.com,
  www.baystatehealth.com/cancer

University of Massachusetts Medical
  School
55 Lake Ave. N
Worcester, MA 01655
508-856-4225
www.umassmed.edu

Michigan

C. S. Mott Children's Hospital
1500 E. Medical Center Drive
L2110 Women's Box 0238
Ann Arbor, MI 48109-0238
734-764-7126
www.cancer.med.umich.edu/clinic/
  pedclinic.htm

Children's Hospital of Michigan
3901 Beaubien Blvd.
Wayne State University
Detroit, MI 48201
313-745-5515
www.childrens-hosp.org

Michigan State University
B220 Clinical Center
East Lansing, MI 48824-1313
517-355-8998
www.msu.edu/unit/phd/

Hurley Medical Center
One Hurley Plaza
Flint, MI 48503-5993
810-762-7303
www.hurleymc.com

DeVos Children's Hospital
100 Michigan NE
Mail Code 85
Grand Rapids, MI 49503-2560
616-391-2086
www.devoschildrens.org

St. John Hospital and Medical Center
Meade Pediatric Hematology/Oncology
19229 Mack Ave., Suite 28
Grosse Point Woods, MI 48236
313-647-3200
www.stjohn.org,
www.vanelslandercancercenter.org/
  ped_oncology.asp

Kalamazoo Center for Medical Studies
601 John St., Suite E-300
Kalamazoo, MI 49007-5341
269-341-6350
www.kcms.msu.edu/pho

William Beaumont Hospital
3577 W. 13 Mile Road
Royal Oak, MI 48073-6769
248-551-0360
www.beaumonthospitals.com

Minnesota

Children's Hospital of Minnesota
2525 Chicago Avenue S., Suite 4150
Minneapolis, MN 55404
612-813-5940
www.childrenshc.org

University of Minnesota Cancer Center
Room D-557 Mayo
420 Delaware St. SE
Minneapolis, MN 55455-0392
612-626-2778
www.cancer.umn.edu/,
    www.cancer.umn.edu/page/clinical/
    pediatric.html

Mayo Clinic and Foundation
200 First St. SW
Rochester, MN 55905-0001
507-284-2511
www.mayo.edu,
www.mayoclinic.org/pediatric-
    hematology-oncology-rst/Minnesota

Mississippi

University of Mississippi Medical Center
    Children's Hospital
2500 N. State Street
Jackson, MS 39216-4505
601-984-5220

Missouri

University of Missouri—Columbia
1 Hospital Dr., 7 W12
Columbia, MO 65212
573-882-3961
www.muhealth.org

Children's Mercy Hospital
2401 Gillham Road
Kansas City, MO 64108
816-234-3265
www.childrens-mercy.org

Cardinal Glennon Children's Hospital
1465 South Grand Blvd.
St. Louis, MO 63104
314-577-5638

Washington University Medical Center
660 S. Euclid Avenue
P.O. Box 8116
St. Louis, MO 63110
314-454-4118

Nebraska

Children's Memorial Hospital of Omaha
8200 Didge Street
Omaha, NE 68114-4113
402-955-3950

University of Nebraska Medical Center
982168 Nebraska Medical Center
Omaha, NE 68198-2168
402-559-7257
www.unmc.edu

Nevada

Nevada Cancer Research Foundation—
    Community Clinical Oncology
    Program
3186 S. Maryland Pkwy
Las Vegas, NV 89109-2306
702-732-0971

New Hampshire

Dartmouth-Hitchcock Medical Center
1 Medical Center Drive
Norris Cotton Cancer Center
Lebanon, NH 03756
603-650-5541
www.hitchcock.org

New Jersey

Hackensack University Medical Center
Tomorrow's Children's Institute
WFAN Pediatric Center, 1st Floor,
  PC 122
Hackensack, NJ 07601
201-996-5437
www.tcikids.com

Saint Barnabas Medical Center
94 Old Short Hills Rd., Suite 182
Livingston, NJ 07039
973-322-2800

Atlantic Health System
Goryeb Children's Hospital
100 Madison Ave., Box 70
Morristown, NJ 07962
973-971-6720

Saint Peter's University Hospital
254 Easton Avenue
New Brunswick, NJ 08901
732-745-6674

University of Medicine and Dentistry of
  New Jersey
Cancer Institute of New Jersey
195 Little Albany Street
New Brunswick, NJ 08901
732-235-5437

Newark Beth Israel Medical Center
201 Lyons Avenue
Newark, NJ 07112-2094
973-926-7161

St. Joseph's Hospital and Medical Center
703 Main St., Xavier 7
Paterson, NJ 07503
973-754-3230
www.stjosephshealth.org

New Mexico

University of New Mexico School of
  Medicine
MSC10 5590
Albuquerque, NM 87131-0001
505-272-4461
www.hsc.unm.edu/pediatrics/
  hematology.shtml

New York

Albany Medical Center
47 New Scotland Avenue
Albany, NY 12208-3419
518-262-5513

Montefiore Medical Center
Section of Pediatric
  Hematology-Oncology
3415 Bainbridge Avenue
Bronx, NY 10467
718-741-2342
www.aecom.yu.edu

Brookdale Hospital Medical Center
One Brookdale Plaza, Suite 346
Brooklyn, NY 11212
718-240-5904

Brooklyn Hospital Center
121 Dekalb Avenue
Brooklyn, NY 11201-5493
718-250-6074
www.tbh.org

Maimonides Medical Center
4802 Tenth Avenue
Brooklyn, NY 11219
718-283-7373

SUNY Health Science Center at
  Brooklyn
450 Clarkson Avenue
Brooklyn, NY 11203-2098
718-270-1693

Roswell Park Cancer Institute
Elm and Carlton Streets
Buffalo, NY 14263
716-845-2333
www.roswellpark.org

Winthrop University Hospital
Division of Pediatric Hematology
200 Old Country Rd., Suite 440
Mineola, NY 11501
516-663-9400

Schneider Children's Hospital
269-01 76th Ave., Room 255
New Hyde Park, NY 11040
718-470-3460

Columbia Presbyterian College of
  Physicians and Surgeons
Pediatric Oncology
161 Fort Washington Ave., I-7
New York, NY 10032-1537
212-305-5808
www.herbertirvingchildren.org

Memorial Sloan Kettering Cancer
  Center
1275 York Avenue
New York, NY 10021-6094
212-639-7951
www.mskcc.org/

Mount Sinai Medical Center
One Gustave L. Levy Place
New York, NY 10029
212-241-7022
www.mssm.edu/peds/
  hematology_oncology/

New York Hospital-Cornell University
  Medical Center
525 E. 68th Street
New York, NY 10021-4885
212-746-3400

New York University Medical Center
550 First Avenue
New York, NY 10016
212-263-6825
www.med.nyu.edu

University of Rochester Medical Center
601 Elmwood Avenue
P.O. Box 777
Rochester, NY 14642
716-275-2981
www.stronghealth.com

State University of New York at Stony
  Brook
HSC T-11, Room 029
Stony Brook, NY 11794-8111
631-444-7720
www.schoolreentry.com

SUNY Upstate Medical University
750 E. Adams Street
Health Science Center
Syracuse, NY 13210
315-464-5294

New York Medical College
Munger Pavillion, Room 110
Valhalla, NY 10595
914-493-7997
www.worldclassmedicine.com/

North Carolina

Mission Hospitals
509 Biltmore Avenue
Asheville, NC 28801-4690
828-213-1111
www.missionhospitals.org

University of North Carolina at Chapel Hill
Division of Hem-Onc CB#7220
Chapel Hill, NC 27599-7220
919-966-1178

Carolinas Medical Center
1000 Blythe Blvd.
Charlotte, NC 28232
704-355-2000

Presbyterian Hospital
200 Hawthorne Lane
P.O. Box 33549
Charlotte, NC 28233
704-384-5227

Duke University Medical Center
Trent Drive
Bell Building, Room 222
Durham, NC 27710
919-684-3401

East Carolina University School of Medicine
200 Moye Blvd.
PCMH - 288W
Greenville, NC 27834
252-744-4676
www.ecu.edu

Wake Forest University School of Medicine
Medical Center Blvd.
Winston-Salem, NC 27157-1081
336-716-4085
www.wfubmc.edu,
www.brennerchildrens.org/

North Dakota

MeritCare Medical Group DBA Roger Maris Cancer Center
820 4th St. N.
Fargo, ND 58122
701-234-7544

Ohio

Children's Hospital Medical Center— Akron
One Perkins Square
Akron, OH 44308-1062
330-543-8730
www.akronchildrens.org/findadoc,
www.akronchildrens.org/depts-services/hematology/

Children's Hospital Medical Center
3333 Burnet Ave., ML-7015
Cincinnati, OH 45229-3039
513-636-4266
www.cincinnatichildrens.org,
www.cincinnatichildrens.org/svc/prog/cancer/default.htm

Children's Hospital at the Cleveland Clinic
9500 Euclid Ave., Desk S20
Cleveland, OH 44195-5217
216-444-5517
www.clevelandclinic.org/pediatrics/departments/cancer_program/cancer_overview.htm,
www.clevelandclinic.org/pediatrics/departments/cancer_program/tumorregistry/

Rainbow Babies and Children's Hospital
11100 Euclid Avenue
Cleveland, OH 44106-5000
216-844-3345
www.rainbowbabies.org/services/specialties/PediatricHematology Oncology/

Columbus Children's Hospital
700 Children's Drive
Columbus, OH 43205-2696
614-722-3552

Children's Hospital Medical Center—
  Dayton
1 Children's Plaza
Dayton, OH 45404-1815
937-641-3111
www.childrensdayton.org,
www.childrensdayton.org/Department/
  hemOnc.htm

Mercy Children's Hospital
2222 Cherry St., Suite 2800
Toledo, OH 43699-0008
419-251-8215
www.mhsnr.org

Toledo Children's Hospital
2142 N. Cove Blvd., 5 South
Toledo, OH 43606
419-291-7815
www.promedica.org

Tod Children's Hospital-Forum Health
500 Gypsy Lane
Medical Education Bldg., 3rd Floor
Youngstown, OH 44501
330-884-3955

Oklahoma

University of Oklahoma Health Sciences
  Center
940 NE 13th Street
Children's Hospital of Oklahoma
Oklahoma City, OK 73104
405-271-5311

Warren Clinic, Inc.
6161 S. Yale Avenue
Tulsa, OK 74136
918-494-2525
www.saintfrancis.com

Oregon

Doernbecher Children's Hospital—
  OHSU
3181 SW Sam Jackson Park Road
Portland, OR 97201-3098
503-494-0714
www.ohsudoernbecher.com/,
  www.ohsu.edu

Emanuel Hospital Health Center
501 N. Graham, Suite 355
Portland, OR 97227
503-281-5053
www.legacyhealth.org/healthcare/
  cancer/childhood.ssi#risk

Pennsylvania

Geisinger Medical Center
100 N. Academy Avenue
Danville, PA 17822-1320
570-271-6848

Penn State Children's Hospital, Hershey
  Medical Center
500 University Dr., H085
Room C7830
Hershey, PA 17033-0850
717-531-6012
www.hmc.psu.edu

Children's Hospital of Philadelphia
324 South 34th Street
Philadelphia, PA 19104-9786
215-590-1000
www.chop.edu

St. Christopher's Hospital for Children
Erie Ave. at Front Street
Philadelphia, PA 19134
215-427-5000
www.stchristophershospital.com

Children's Hospital of Pittsburgh
3705 Fifth Avenue
Pittsburgh, PA 15213-2583
412-692-5055
www.chp.edu/clinical/
   03a_hemato.php?base=hema

Rhode Island

Rhode Island Hospital
593 Eddy Street
MPS-1
Providence, RI 02903
401-444-5171

South Carolina

Medical University of South Carolina
135 Rutledge Avenue
P.O. Box 250558
Charleston, SC 29425
843-792-2957
www.musckids.com

South Carolina Cancer Center
7 Richland Medical Park, Suite 203
Columbia, SC 29203-6897
803-434-3533
www.palmettohealth.org

Children's Hospital of the Greenville
   Hospital System
900 West Faris Road
Greenville, SC 29605
803-455-8898

South Dakota

Sioux Valley Children's Specialty Clinics
1305 W. 18th Street
Sioux Falls, SD 57117-5039
605-333-7171
www.siouxvalley.org

Tennessee

T. C. Thompson Children's Hospital
910 Blackford Street
Chattanooga, TN 37403
423-778-7289
www.erlanger.org

East Tennessee State University
ETSU Cancer Center
400 N. State of Franklin Road
Johnson City, TN 37604
423-433-6200

East Tennessee Children's Hospital
2018 Clinch Ave. SW
P.O. Box 15010
Knoxville, TN 37916
865-541-8266
www.etch.com

St. Jude Children's Research Hospital
   Memphis
332 N. Lauderdale
Memphis, TN 38105
901-495-3300
www.stjude.org

Vanderbilt Children's Hospital
2220 Pierce Avenue
397 PRB
Nashville, TN 37232-6310
615-936-1762
www.vanderbiltchildrens.com,
   www.vanderbiltchildrens.com/cancer

Texas

Texas Tech UHSC—Amarillo
1400 Coulter
Amarillo, TX 79106
806-354-5527
www.ama.ttuhsc.edu

Children's Hospital of Austin
One Children's Place
1400 North IH 35
Austin, TX 78701
512-324-8480

Driscoll Children's Hospital
3533 South Alameda
Corpus Christi, TX 78411-1721
512-694-5311
www.driscollchildrens.org,
    www.driscollchildrens.org/oncology/

North Texas Hospital for Children at
    Medical City Dallas
7777 Forest Lane, D-400
Dallas, TX 75230
972-566-6647
www.ntxhospitalforchildren.com

University of Texas Southwestern
    Medical Center
Pediatrics Department
5323 Harry Hines Blvd.
Dallas, TX 75390-9063
214-456-2382
www.childrens.com/ccbd

Cook Children's Medical Center
901 Seventh Ave., Suite 220
Fort Worth, TX 76104-9958
817-885-4020
www.cookchildrens.org

University of Texas Medical Branch
301 University Blvd., Rt. 0361
Galveston, TX 77555-0361
409-772-2341

M. D. Anderson Cancer Center
1515 Holcombe Blvd.
P.O. Box 87
Houston, TX 77030-4095
713-792-6620
www.mdanderson.org/

Texas Children's Cancer Center at Baylor
    College of Medicine
6621 Fannin St., MC 1410.00
Houston, TX 77030-2399
832-824-4200
www.txccc.org

Wilford Hall Medical Center
2200 Bergquist Dr., Suite 1
Wilford Hall Medical Center
Lackland AFB, TX 78236-5300
210-292-5684

Children's Hem/Onc Team, Covenant
    Children's Hospital
3606 21st St., Suite 304
Lubbock, TX 79410
806-725-4840

Methodist Children's Hospital of South
    Texas
7711 Louis Pasteur Dr., Suite 306
San Antonio, TX 78229-3993
210-614-4011
www.sahealth.com

University of Texas Health Science
    Center at San Antonio
8th Floor, Mail Code 7810
333 N. Santa Rosa
San Antonio, TX 78207
210-704-3405
www.pediatricsuthscsa.edu

Scott & White Memorial Hospital
2401 S. 31st Street
Temple, TX 76508
254-724-2006
www.sw.org

Utah

Primary Children's Medical Center
100 N. Medical Dr., Suite 1400
Salt Lake City, UT 84113-1100
801-588-2680
www.ihc.com/primary/

Vermont

University of Vermont College of
    Medicine
Given Medical Building, Room E203
Burlington, VT 05405
802-847-2850

Virginia

University of Virginia Health Sciences
    Center
Pediatric Oncology
P.O. Box 386
Charlottesville, VA 22908
804-924-5105

Inova Fairfax Hospital
8301 Arlington Blvd., Suite 209
Fairfax, VA 22031
703-876-9111

Children's Hospital—King's Daughters
601 Children's Lane
Norfolk, VA 23507-1971
757-668-7243

Naval Medical Center/Portsmouth
    (USOC)
620 John Paul Jones Circle
Portsmouth, VA 23708-2197
757-953-4522
www.nmcp.mar.med.navy.mil/
    Pediatrics/hemeonc.asp

Virginia Commonwealth University
    Health System—Medical College of
    Virginia
P.O. Box 980121
Richmond, VA 23298-0121
804-828-9605

Carilion Medical Center for Children at
    Roanoke Community Hospital
101 Elm Ave., 5th Floor
Roanoke, VA 24029
540-985-8055
www.carilion.com

Washington

Children's Hospital and Regional
    Medical Center
CHRMC, Mailstop: 6D-1
4800 Sand Point Way NE
Seattle, WA 98105
206-987-2106
www.seattlechildrens.org

Sacred Heart Children's Hospital
101 W. 8th Avenue
P.O. Box 2555
Spokane, WA 99220-2555

Madigan Army Medical Center (USOC)
Fitzsimmons Dr., Bldg. 9040
Tacoma, WA 98431
253-968-1980

Mary Bridge Hospital
311 South L Street
P.O. Box 5299
Tacoma, WA 98405
253-403-3481

West Virginia

West Virginia University HSC—
    Charleston
830 Pennsylvania Avenue
Charleston, WV 25302
304-388-1540

Cabell Huntington Hospital
1600 Medical Center Drive
Huntington, WV 25701
304-691-1300

West Virginia University HSC—
   Morgantown
P.O. Box 9214
Health Sciences N.
Morgantown, WV 26506
304-293-1217

Wisconsin

St. Vincent Hospital—Wisconsin
835 S. Van Buren Street
Green Bay, WI 54301
920-433-8889
www.stvincenthospital.org

University of Wisconsin Children's
   Hospital—Madison
600 Highland Avenue
Dept. of Pediatric Hem-Onc
Madison, WI 53792-0001
608-263-6200
www.uwchildrenshospital.org,
   www.outlook-life.org/

Marshfield Clinic
1000 N. Oak Avenue
Marshfield, WI 54449-5772
715-387-5511
www.marshfieldclinic.org,
   http://research.marshfieldclinic.org/

Midwest Children's Cancer Center
8701 Watertown Plank Road
MACC Fund Research Center
Milwaukee, WI 53226
414-456-4170

Wellness Resources

American Association for Music
   Therapy
P.O. Box 80012
Valley Forge, PA 19484
215-265-5467

American Physical Therapy Association
111 North Fairfax Street
Alexandria, VA 22314
800-999-APTA
www.APTA.org

American Speech-Language Hearing
   Association
www.asha.org

The Anderson Network (telephone
   support for patients and their
   families)
800-345-6324
www.mdacc.tmc.edu/~andnet

Brain Injury Association
www.biusa.org

The Cancer Hot Line, R. A. Bloch Cancer
   Foundation (matches patients with
   other brain tumor survivors)
800-433-0464
www.blochcancer.org

Cancervive
6500 Wilshire Blvd., Suite 500
Los Angeles, CA 90048
310-203-9232
www.cancervive.org

CANHELP
P.O. Box 103
32220 Rainier Ave. NE
Port Gamble, WA 98364
800-565-1732
www.canhelp.com

Commission on Accreditation of
  Rehabilitation Facilities
4891 East Grant Road
Tucson, AZ 85712
520-325-1044
www.carf.org

Connections (pen pal program for
  patients and their families)
American Brain Tumor Association
2720 River Road
Des Plaines, IL 60018
800-886-2282
www.abta.org

Dana-Farber Cancer Institute One to
  One: The Cancer Connection
  (matches patients with the same
  diagnosis)
617-632-4880

George Washington University Health
  Resource Center
www.health.gwu.edu

Guardian Brain Foundation
www.guardianbrain.com

Hydrocephalus Association
www.hydroassoc.org

Independent Living Research Utilization
2323 South Shepard, Suite 1000
Houston, TX 77019
713-520-0232
www.ilru.org

Learning Services Corporation
3710 University Dr., Suite 201
Durham, NC 27707
800-888-REHAB
www.learningservices.com

National Aphasia Association
www.aphasia.org

National Center for Learning
  Disabilities, Inc.
www.ncld.org

National Institute on Deafness and
  Other Communication Disorders
www.nidcd.nih.gov

National Center for Complementary
  and Alternative Medicine at the
  National Institutes of Health
www.nccam.nih.gov

The Wellness Community
www.wellnesscommunity.org

Tim and Tom Gullikson Foundation
  (college scholarship program)
Chicago, Illinois
888-GULLIKSON
www.gulliksonfoundation.org

General Resources for Patients with Brain Tumors

The American Cancer Society
1599 Clifton Rd. NE
Atlanta, GA 30329
800-227-2345
www.cancer.org

American Brain Tumor Association
2720 River Road
Des Plaines, IL 60018
800-886-2282
www.abta.org

Brainlife (brain tumor medical
database)
www.brainlife.org

The Brain Science Foundation
277 Linden Street
Suite 207
Wellesley, MA 02482
866-492-2466
www.brainsciencefoundation.org

Brain Tumor Foundation
1350 Avenue of the Americas, Suite 1200
New York, NY 10019
212-265-2401
www.braintumorfoundation.org

Brain Tumour Foundation of Canada
620 Colborne St., Suite 301
London, Ontario, Canada N6B 3R0
519-642-7725
www.braintumour.ca

The Brain Tumor Society
124 Watertown St., Suite 3H
Watertown, MA 02472-2500
800-770-8287
www.tbts.org

Canadian Cancer Society
www.cancer.ca

Cancer Consultants
www.cancerconsultants.com

The Healing Exchange: Brain Trust
186 Hampshire Street
Cambridge, MA 02139-1320
877-252-8480
www.braintrust.org

The Musella Foundation
musella@virtualtrials.com

The National Brain Tumor Foundation
323 Geary St., Suite 510
San Francisco, CA 94102
800-934-2873
www.braintumor.org

The National Cancer Institute
www.cancernet.nci.nih.gov

The National Coalition for Cancer
Survivorship
1010 Wayne Avenue
Silver Spring, MD 20910-0560
301-650-9127
www.cansearch.org

National Institutes of Health
Office of Cancer Communications
National Cancer Institute
Bldg. 31, #10A29
Bethesda, MD 20205
301-496-6631
www.nci.nih.gov

National Institute of Neurologic
Disorders and Stroke (NINDS)
31 Center Drive
Bldg. 31, #8A06, MSC-2540
Bethesda, MD 20892-2540
800-352-9424
www.ninds.nih.gov

North American Brain Tumor Coalition
www.nabraintumor.org

Oncolink
www.oncolink.com

WebMD Health
www.mywebmd.com

Opportunities to Support Brain Tumor Research

Many foundations and other funds provide the opportunity to support research in brain tumors. They include:

American Brain Tumor Association
2720 River Road
Des Plaines, IL 60018
800-886-2282
www.abta.org

Brain Science Foundation
277 Linden St., Suite 207
Welesley, MA 02482
www.brainsciencefoundation.org

The Brain Tumor Society
124 Watertown St., Suite 3H
Watertown, MA 02472-2500
800-770-8287
www.tbts.org

The National Brain Tumor Foundation
323 Geary St., Suite 510
San Francisco, CA 94102
800-934-2873
www.braintumor.org

Peter Black Research Fund
Department of Neurosurgery
Brigham and Women's Hospital
75 Francis Street
Boston, MA 02115
www.blacklab.org

Florida Brain Tumor Association
P.O. Box 770182
Coral Springs, FL 33077-0182
www.fbta.info

ACKNOWLEDGMENTS

■

Many people have contributed to this book: my patients, who have taught me enormously; my family, Katharine, Dia, Libby, Katy, Peter Thomas, and Christopher, who have tolerated my hours away from home taking care of patients; my trainees, who have continued to teach me year by year whether as residents, fellows, or colleagues; my present and past coworkers, especially Alexandra Golby, Mark Johnson, Elizabeth Claus, John Park, Patrick Wen, Naren Ramakrishna, Jay Loeffler, Howard Fine, Stephanie Weiss, Caryn Rhouddou, Donna Dello Iacono, Nancy Olsen Bailey, Kwan Quach, Shelly Russell, Maria Gonzalez, Sandi Rufo, Heather Galvin Carter, Chuck Stiles, Matthew Larkin, Jeff Pike, Tim Lynch, Nicole Fein, Janice Fairhurst, and all the health-care workers who have contributed to our patient care.

Many friends have helped immensely in our research efforts in brain tumors. I particularly want to thank Kathleen and Steven Haley, Kristin O'Sullivan, and the Brain Science Foundation for helping to create the Meningioma Center at the Brigham and Women's Hospital and supporting its work; and Tom and Jean Hagerty for their support of the Glioma Center. Without their help this book would not have been conceived.

Several colleagues have been kind enough to read and modify the text: Donna Dello Iacono, Nancy Olsen Bailey, Lisa Doherty, Rachel Silverman, nurses in the Dana-Farber/Brigham and Women's Cancer Center brain tumor group; Tish Reidy, nurse practitioner at Children's Hospital Boston; Paul Faircloth and Ellen Golden, licensed social workers at Brigham and Women's Hospital; Doctors David Rosenthal, Mark Johnson, Christopher Turner, Mark Kieran, Stephanie Weiss, Liliana Goumnerova, Scott Pomeroy, Patrick Wen, Jan Drappatz, Malcolm Rogers, Gerald Koocher, and Mark Rockoff, who have read and commented on chapters appropriate to their areas of expertise; and the many patients who were willing to share their experiences and make comments.

I wish to thank Julie Levesque for her line drawings and Dr. Liangge Hsu for many of the MRI images used in this book.

Kit Ward and Supurna Banerjee were extremely helpful in the editing process. Above all, however, Sharon Hogan was crucial in creating the first drafts of the book and gently prodded to get it done. Without her, this book may never have seen the light of day.

INDEX

—■—

surgery *(cont.)*
  preoperative visit, 136–37, 231–32
  preparing for your planned, 133–38
  for primary tumors, 43–44, 49, 52–53, 55, 56, 58, 60, 61, 62, 63, 66–67, 68, 69, 72, 74
  pros and cons of, 87–88
  radiosurgery, *see* radiosurgery
  recovery from, 245–49
  relationship with your surgeon, 132–33
  removal of whole tumor vs. biopsy, 139–40
  risks and complications, 148–52, 234
  terminology, 139
  transsphenoidal procedures, 67
  types of, 139–40
  see also specific types of brain tumors
swallowing, difficulty, 79
  therapy for, 246
swelling of the brain, *see* cerebral swelling (edema)
symptoms and signs, 17–20, 127
  see also specific symptoms and individual types of brain tumors

targeted molecular therapies, 195–97
tarseva, 157
teenagers, *see* childhood and adolescence, brain tumors found in; raising a child with a brain tumor
temozolomide (Methazolastone, Temodar), 157, 180, 182, 183, 184, 187, 195
tentorial notch, 42
tentorium, 14
thalamus, 9, 12
Thomas, Dylan, 263–64
3D conformal radiation (3DCRT), 159, 160–62
thyroid hormone, 174, 236
TM-601, 157
TOPS (Teens of Parent Survivors), 101
translational research, 201, 202, 265
transsphenoidal operation, 49
treatment options, 123–240
  alternative and complementary therapies, 129, 183, 252–59
  for children, 228–40
  determination of, 39, 86–87
  early, 19–20, 35
  outline of decisions regarding, 87
  pros and cons of different types of, 87–88
  resources, 280–309
  withdrawal of treatment, *see* supportive care
  see also specific options, e.g., chemotherapy; radiation therapy; surgery; watching and waiting; *and specific types of tumors*
Trilogy system of radiosurgery, 165
tuberous sclerosis, 7
tumor suppressor genes, 8, 41
Turcot's syndrome, 6
Turner, Dr. Christopher, 113, 229
types of brain tumors, 35–79

cell type, classification by, 38
Karnofsky performance score (KPS), 39
tumor grade, 38–39

uniqueness of each case, 85, 86, 263
urinalysis, 136
urologists, 247

vagus nerve stimulator, 21
vascular endothelial growth factor receptor (VEGF) inhibitors, 196
vascular malformation, 18
ventriculo-peritoneal (VP) shunt, 151
vertigo (dizziness), 51
vestibular schwannomas (acoustic neuromas), 19, 36, 49–54, 126
  diagnosis of, 51
  symptoms of, 51
  treatment of, 51–53, 262
vincristine (Oncovin), 179, 182
vision
  double (diplopia), 19, 35, 42, 67, 73, 74, 79, 229
  eye tests, 48
  loss of, 17, 19, 47, 56, 66, 229
  problems, generally, 57, 60, 66, 247
visual field tests (perimetry), 31
visualization, 256
vitamin and mineral supplements, 168–69, 253
vomiting, *see* nausea and vomiting
Von Hippel-Landau disease, 69

waiting room, informing family of surgery's progress in, 137–38, 234
watching and waiting, 125–31, 261–62
  after initial treatment, 126–27
  as the first steps in treatment, 126
  life decisions while, 129–30
  primary tumors and, 43, 52, 56, 58, 61, 63, 66, 126
  priorities, reassessing, 130–31
  regular MRI scans, what to expect from, 128–29
  signs and symptoms to monitor, 127
  strategies for coping, 127–28
weakness, 19, 57, 60, 63, 71, 79, 150
Web sites, *see* Internet, responsible information sources on the
whole-brain radiation, 78, 159, 160
wigs, 172, 186
withdrawal of treatment, *see* supportive care
work
  insurance coverage, *see* health insurance
  possible effects of brain tumor on, 102–103
  preparing for surgery and, 134
World Health Organization, 38

Yeats, William Butler, 129
yoga, 256

About the Authors

DR. PETER M. BLACK is the Franc D. Ingraham Professor of Neurosurgery at Harvard Medical School and chair of the Departments of Neurosurgery at Brigham and Women's Hospital and Children's Hospital Boston. He is also the chief of neurosurgical oncology at the Dana-Farber Cancer Institute. He has devoted his professional life to caring for patients with neurosurgical disorders, especially brain tumors, hydrocephalus, and epilepsy; teaching students, residents, fellows, and other neurosurgeons; working with neurosurgeons from other countries, and doing research to improve future care for patients with brain tumors. He is continuously grateful for the support of his family, coworkers, patients, and colleagues.

SHARON CLOUD HOGAN is a writer and editor who specializes in working with physicians to develop accessible books for the general public. In addition to her work as a collaborator on several medical books, she is the coauthor of *The Art of Civilized Conversation* and *Teach Your Dog to Read*. She is also an editor at *The New England Journal of Medicine* in Boston.